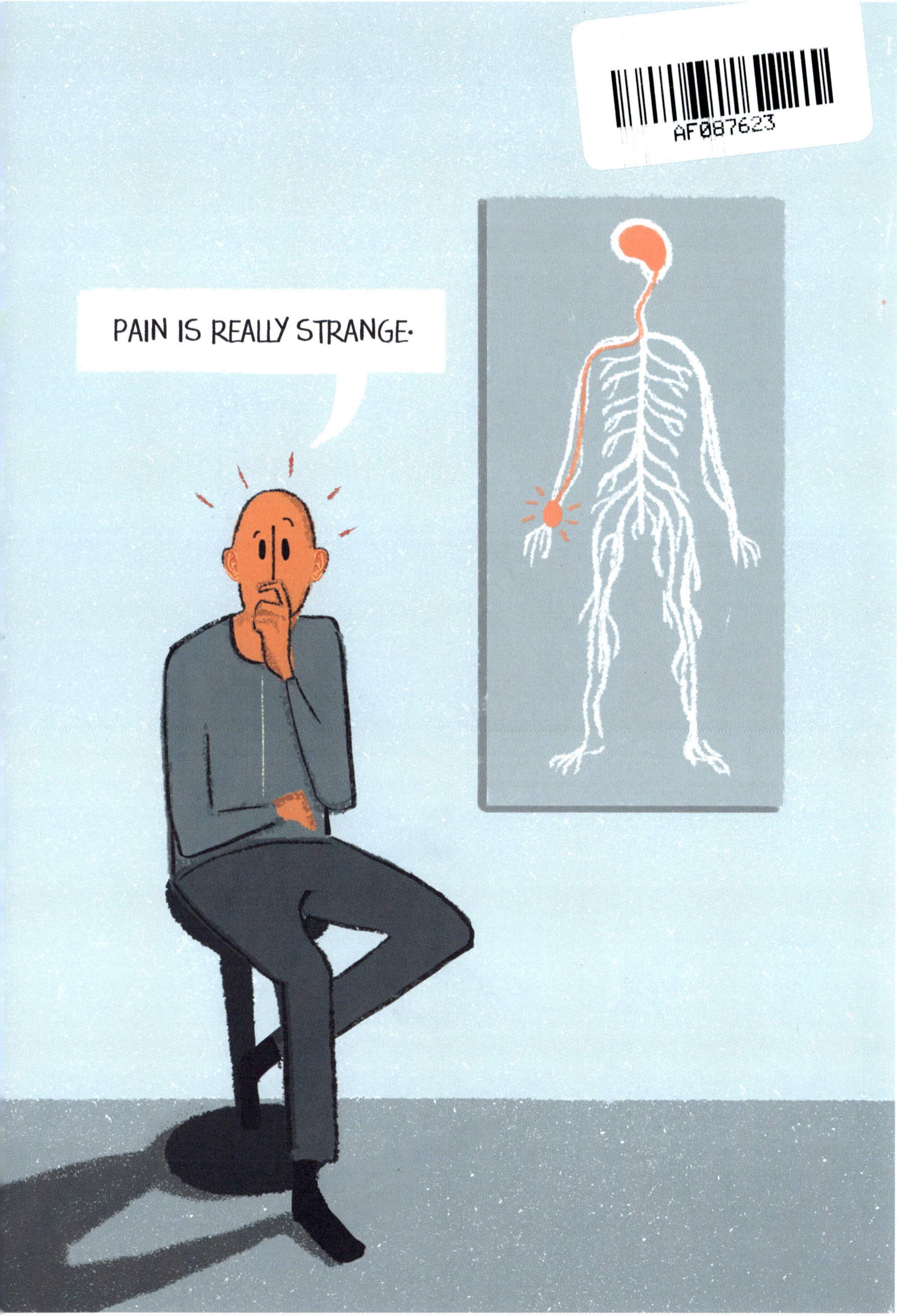
PAIN IS REALLY STRANGE.

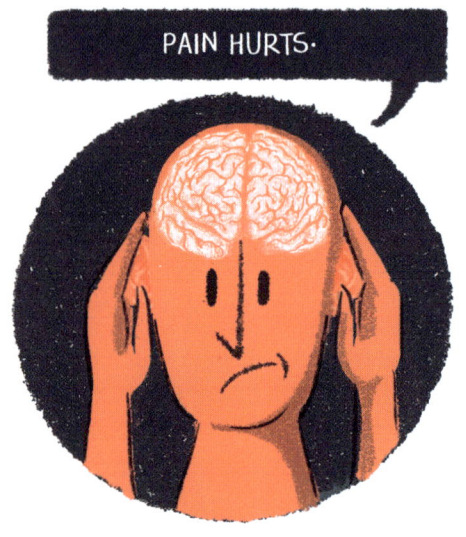

PAIN HURTS.

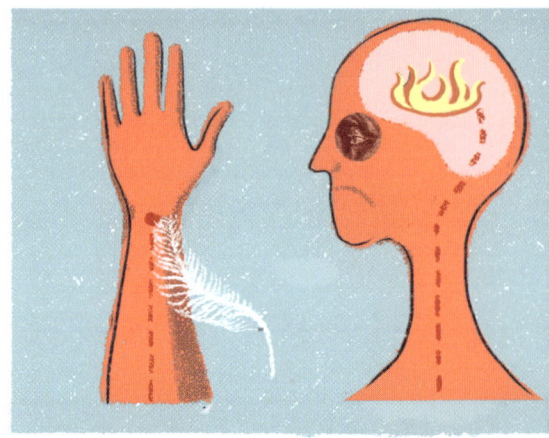

A YOUNG DANCER SPRAINS HER WRIST AND THE PAIN AMPLIFIES UNTIL BEING TOUCHED WITH A FEATHER IS A TERRIFYING BURNING.

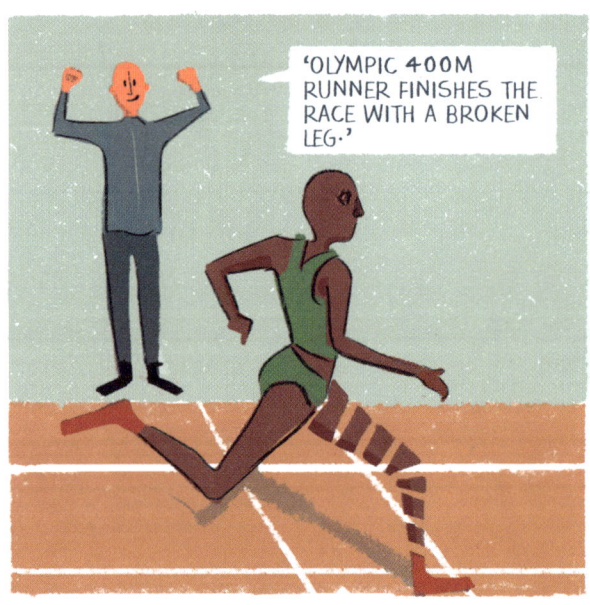

'OLYMPIC 400M RUNNER FINISHES THE RACE WITH A BROKEN LEG.'

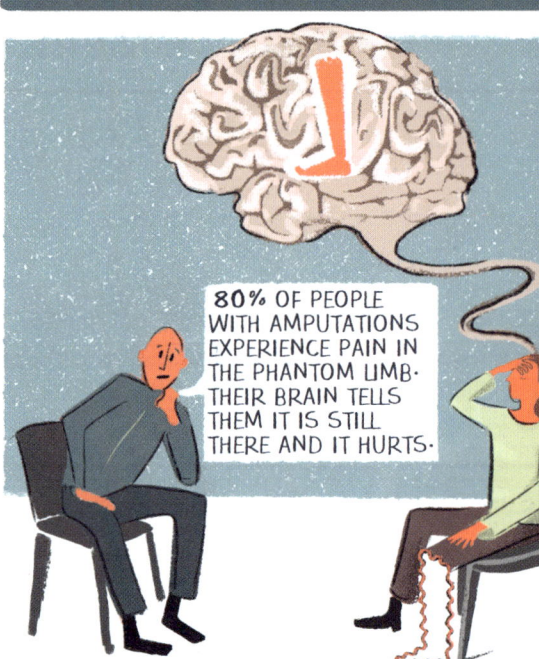

80% OF PEOPLE WITH AMPUTATIONS EXPERIENCE PAIN IN THE PHANTOM LIMB. THEIR BRAIN TELLS THEM IT IS STILL THERE AND IT HURTS.

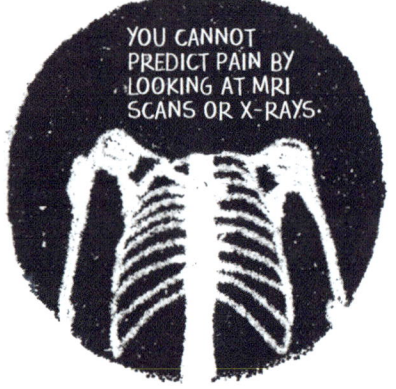

YOU CANNOT PREDICT PAIN BY LOOKING AT MRI SCANS OR X-RAYS.

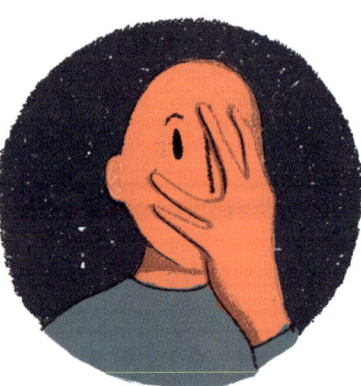

SEEING X-RAYS AND MRI SCANS MAY ACTUALLY MAKE YOU MORE LIKELY TO EXPERIENCE PAIN AS THEY LOOK SCARY.

IN FACT MANY OF US HAVE TORN TISSUES, DISC BULGES AND KNARLY LOOKING BONES WITH NO PAIN.

 In the London 2012 Olympics Manteo Mitchell ran the first leg of the heat for the 4x400 metres relay and felt a pop. X-rays revealed afterwards that he broke his left fibula. His team still qualified (Huffington Post 2012).

The dancer's experience is the centre of a great TED talk by (2011). 'Allodynia' is the term for when light touch generates pain - the nervous system is confused and sensitized.

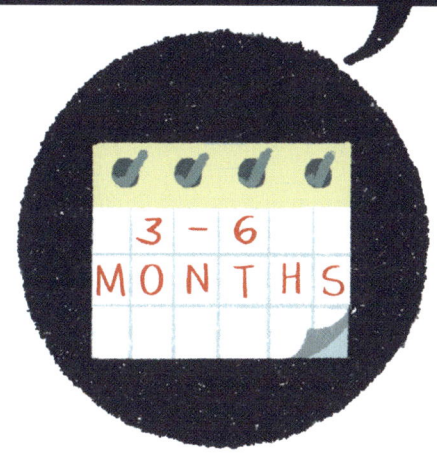
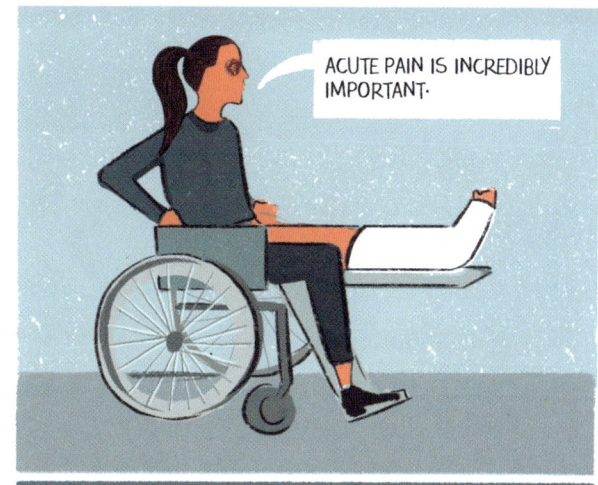
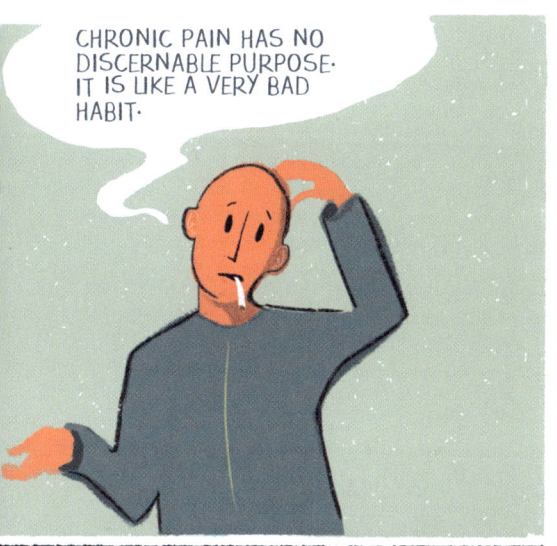
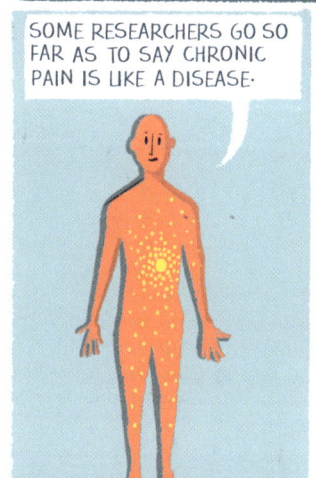
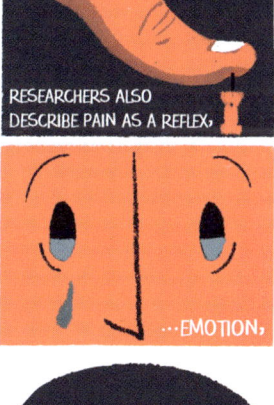
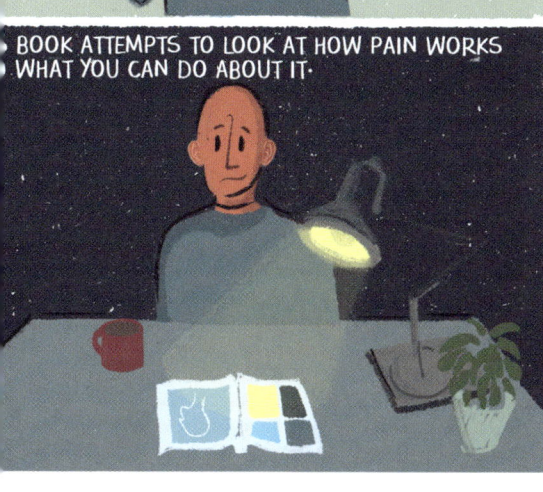
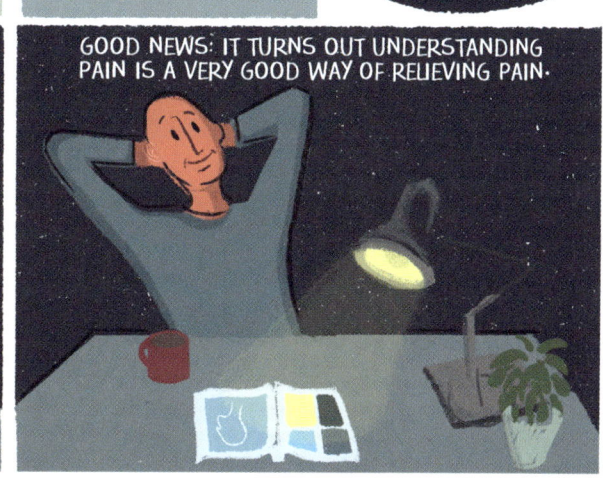

is a disease' (Krane 2011). Pain as 'unresolved emotional trauma held the body' (Levine and Phillips 2012). '...emerging concepts of aptive pain and fear suggest that they share basic neuronal circuits and r mechanisms of memory formation' (Sandkühler and Lee 2013).

Reading a big Lancet study on pain education was the inspiration for this book. Michaleff et al (2014) compared interventions for chronic whiplash sufferers. 30 mins of reading on understanding pain and how the nervous system worked, plus 2 phone calls performed as well as 20(!) sessions of physiotherapy. Yowser.

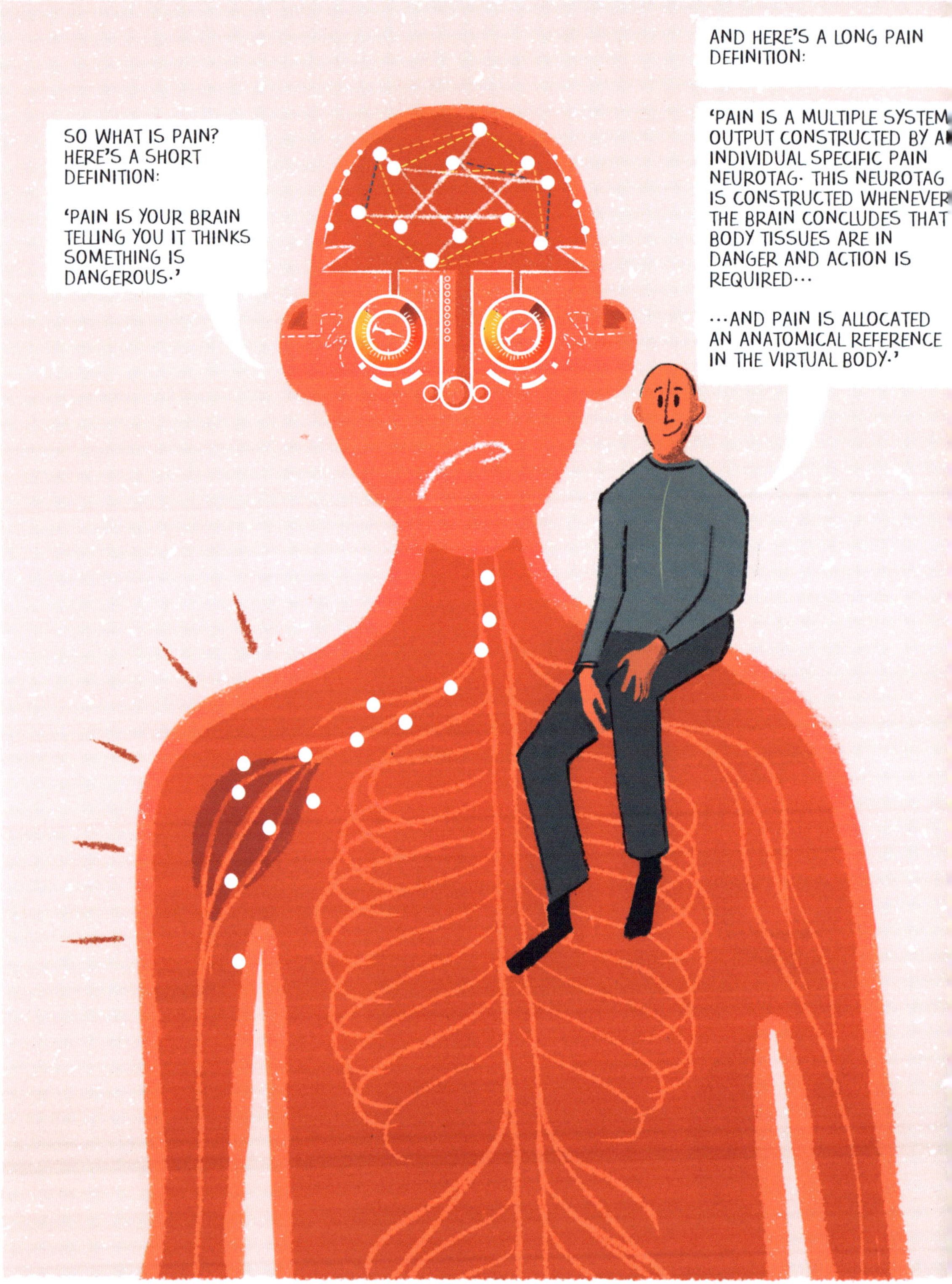

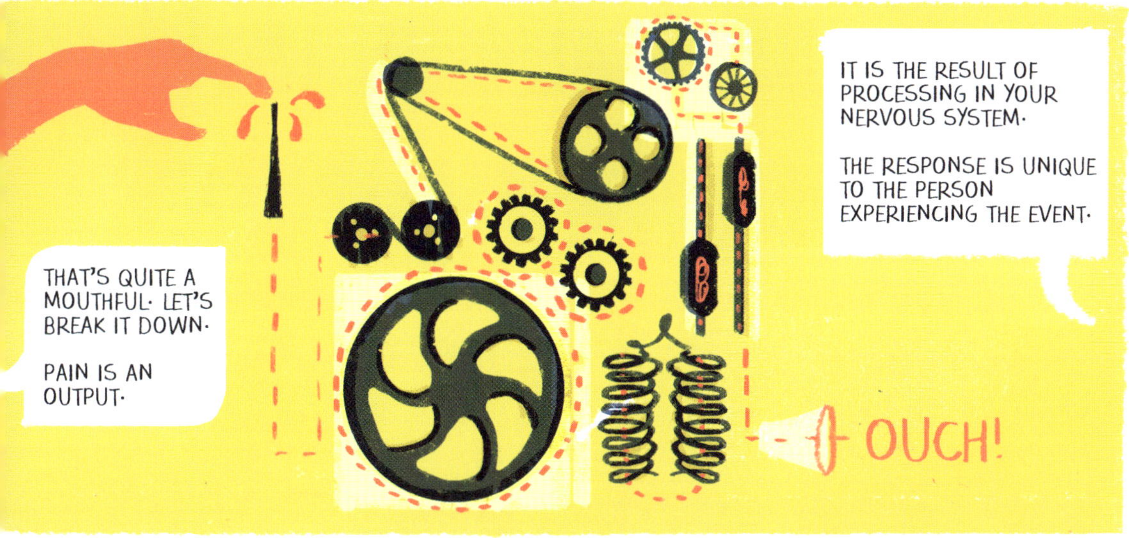
THAT'S QUITE A MOUTHFUL. LET'S BREAK IT DOWN.
PAIN IS AN OUTPUT.
IT IS THE RESULT OF PROCESSING IN YOUR NERVOUS SYSTEM.
THE RESPONSE IS UNIQUE TO THE PERSON EXPERIENCING THE EVENT.
OUCH!

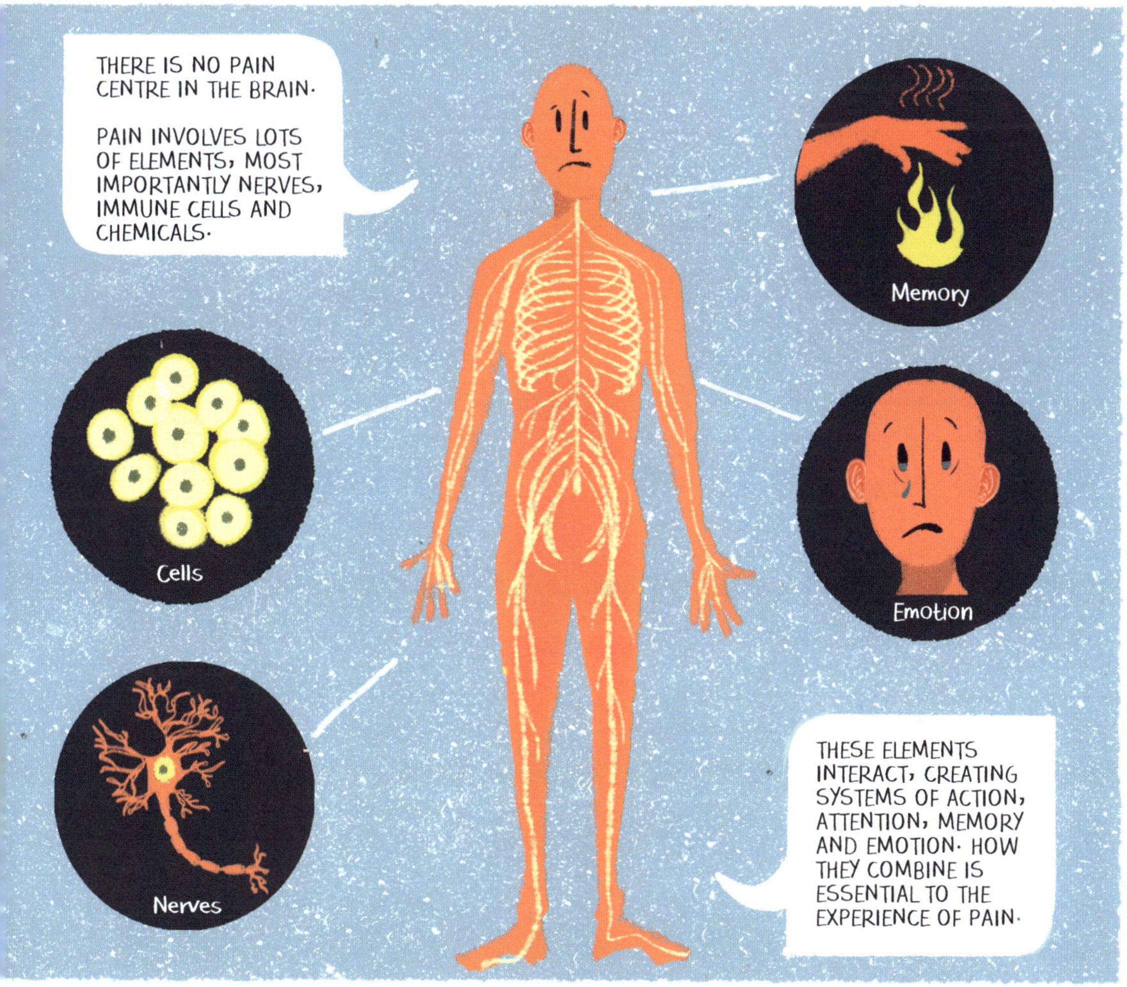
THERE IS NO PAIN CENTRE IN THE BRAIN.
PAIN INVOLVES LOTS OF ELEMENTS, MOST IMPORTANTLY NERVES, IMMUNE CELLS AND CHEMICALS.
Memory
Cells
Emotion
Nerves
THESE ELEMENTS INTERACT, CREATING SYSTEMS OF ACTION, ATTENTION, MEMORY AND EMOTION. HOW THEY COMBINE IS ESSENTIAL TO THE EXPERIENCE OF PAIN.

The long definition is taken from the leading pain researcher Lorimer Moseley (2003). I have changed 'neurosignature' to the shorter 'neurotag'.

Moseley in his talks and writing often states that the brain is evaluating 'How dangerous is this really?' Pain is the answer if the brain decides something is dangerous.

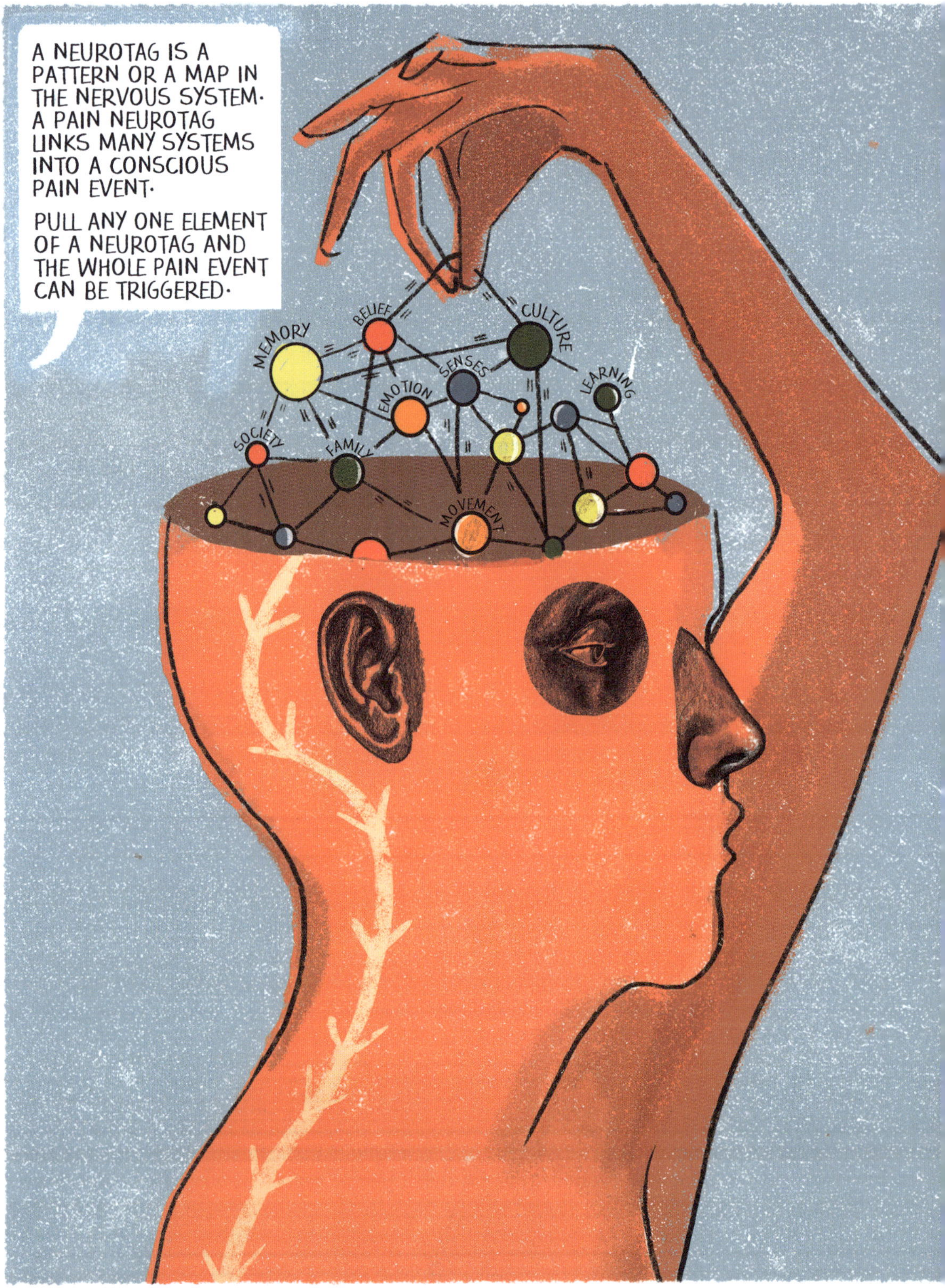
A NEUROTAG IS A PATTERN OR A MAP IN THE NERVOUS SYSTEM. A PAIN NEUROTAG LINKS MANY SYSTEMS INTO A CONSCIOUS PAIN EVENT.
PULL ANY ONE ELEMENT OF A NEUROTAG AND THE WHOLE PAIN EVENT CAN BE TRIGGERED.
MEMORY
BELIEF
CULTURE
SENSES
EMOTION
LEARNING
SOCIETY
FAMILY
MOVEMENT

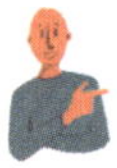

'We can think of pain as a conscious experience that emerges in response to activity in a particular network of brain cells that are spread across the brain. We can call the network a "neurotag" and we can call the brain cells th make up the neurotag "member brain cells"' (Moseley 2012b).

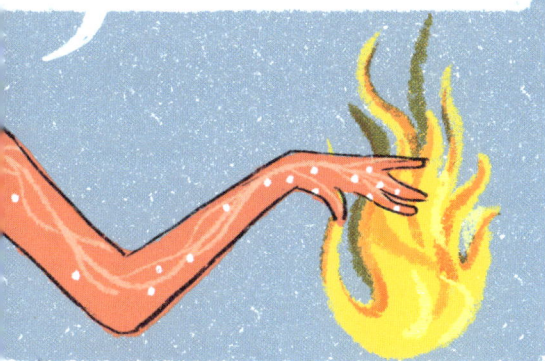
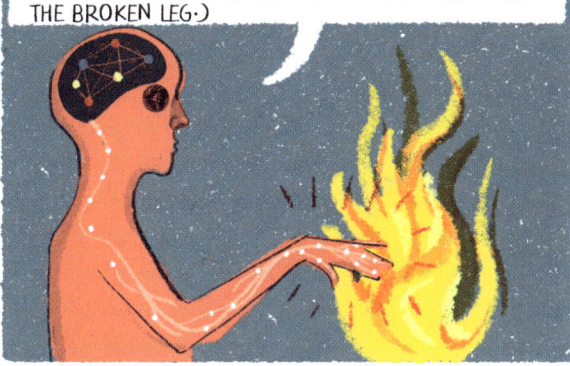
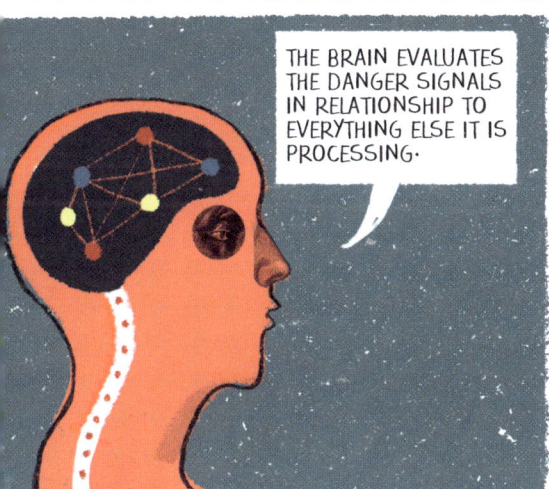
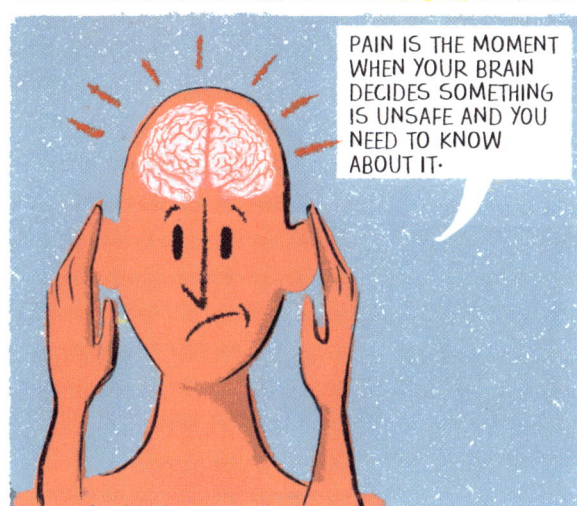
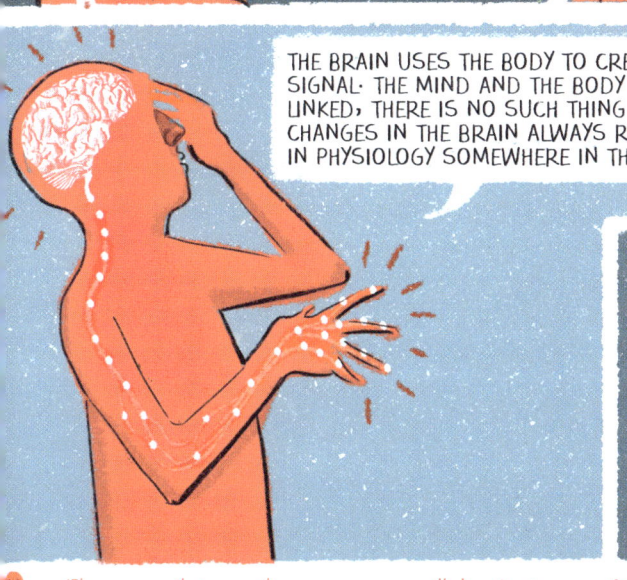

'The neurons that carry those messages are called nociceptors, or danger receptors. We call the system that detects and transmits noxious events "nociception".

Critically, nociception is neither sufficent nor necessary for pain. But most of the time pain is associated with some nociception' (Moseley 2012b).

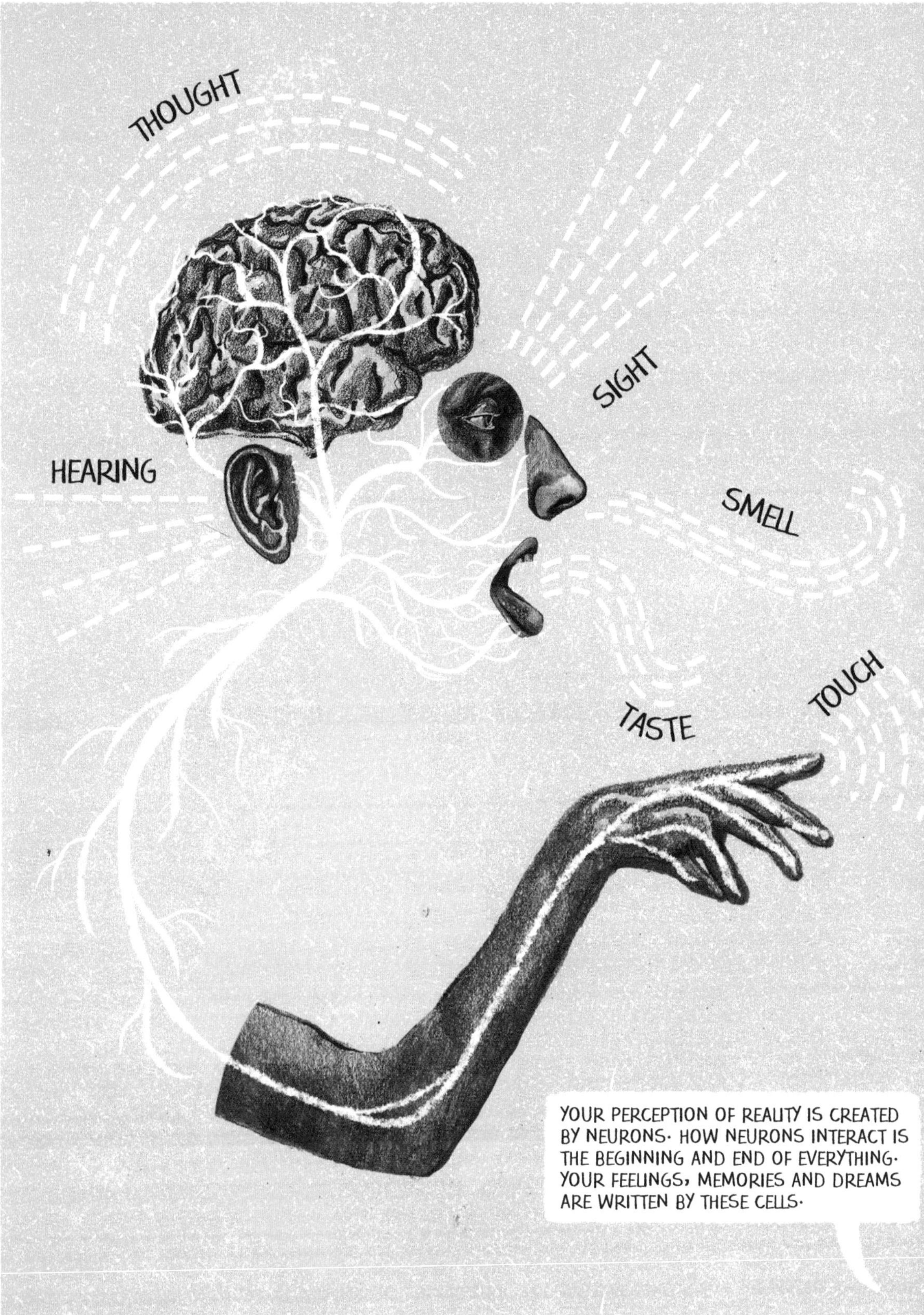
THOUGHT
SIGHT
HEARING
SMELL
TASTE
TOUCH
YOUR PERCEPTION OF REALITY IS CREATED BY NEURONS. HOW NEURONS INTERACT IS THE BEGINNING AND END OF EVERYTHING. YOUR FEELINGS, MEMORIES AND DREAMS ARE WRITTEN BY THESE CELLS.

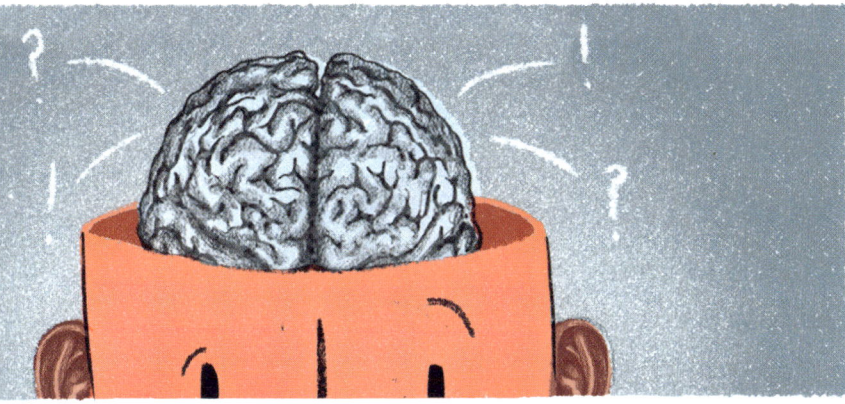

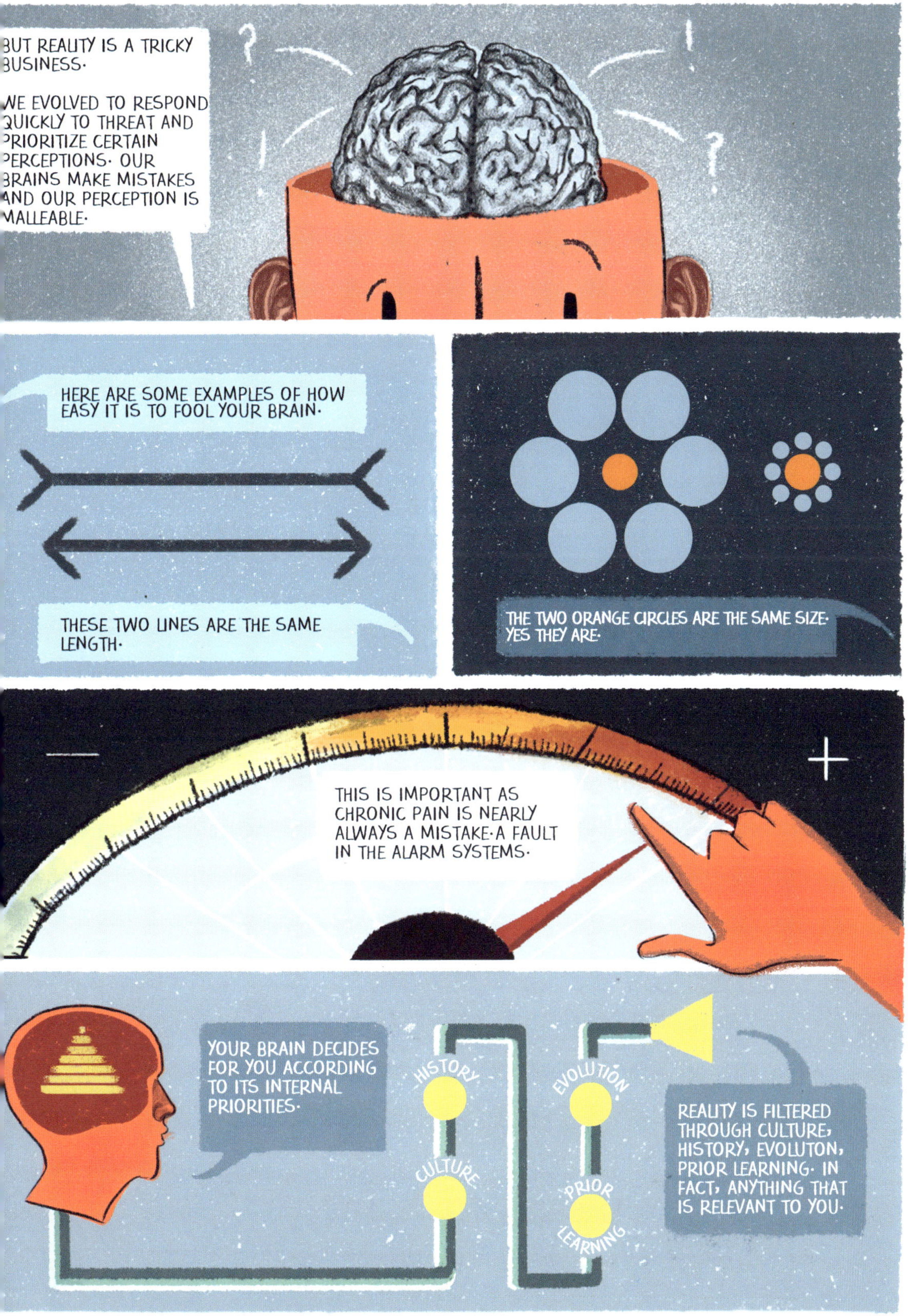

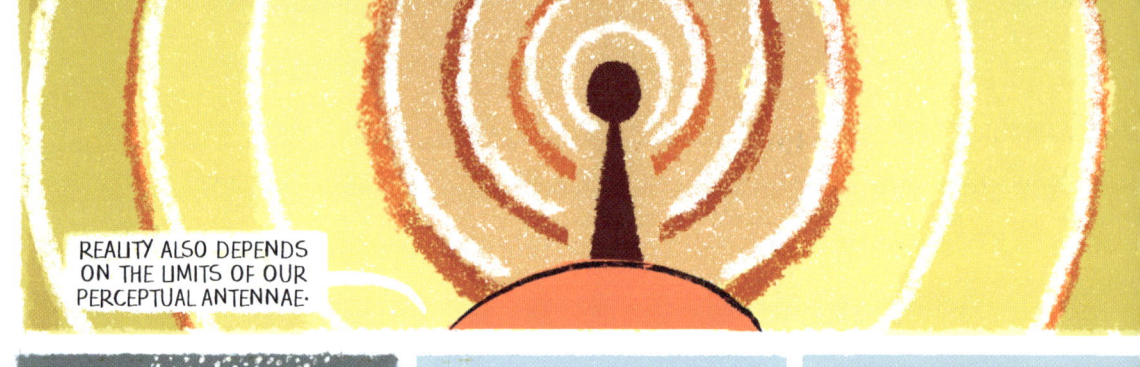

REALITY ALSO DEPENDS ON THE LIMITS OF OUR PERCEPTUAL ANTENNAE.

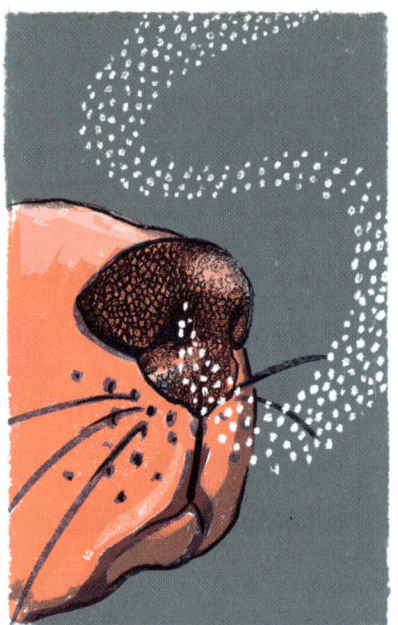

YOU CANNOT SMELL WHAT A DOG SMELLS.

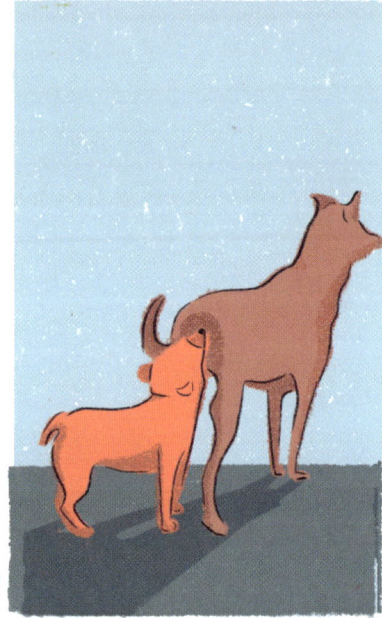

THAT IS OFTEN A GOOD THING.

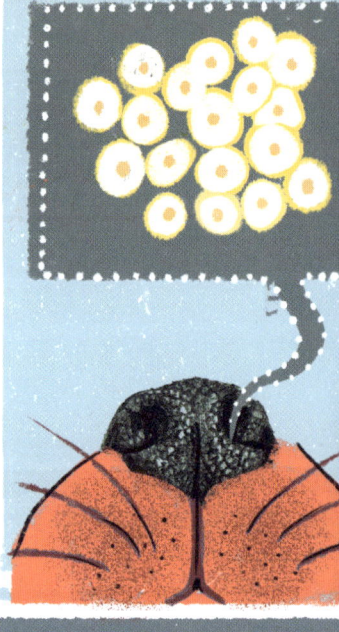

SOME DOGS CAN SMELL CANCER OR EPILEPSY. THAT WOULD BE QUITE USEFUL.

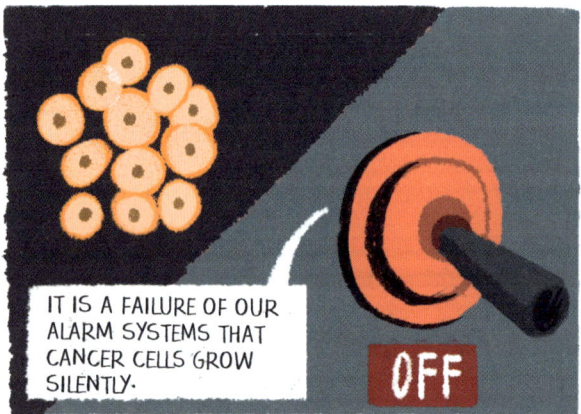

IT IS A FAILURE OF OUR ALARM SYSTEMS THAT CANCER CELLS GROW SILENTLY.

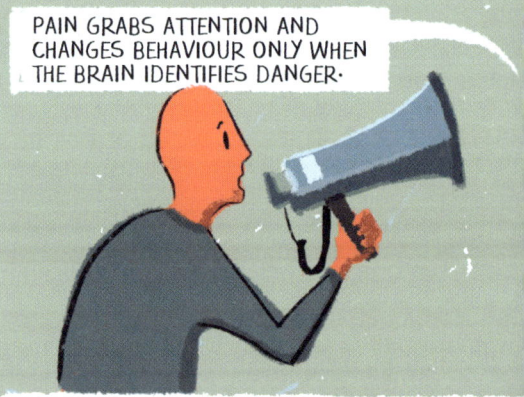

PAIN GRABS ATTENTION AND CHANGES BEHAVIOUR ONLY WHEN THE BRAIN IDENTIFIES DANGER.

Dogs 'sniff out prostate cancer with 98% accuracy' (Medical News Today 2014). 'Reports suggest that some dogs can be trained to anticipate epileptic seizures' (Kirton et al 2008).

Two causes of chronic pain are known to involve more than sensitiza Cancer pain is often intractable and emerges when tumours grow continuously compress surrounding structures. Neuropathic pain, w the nerve structure is damaged, is also a special case.

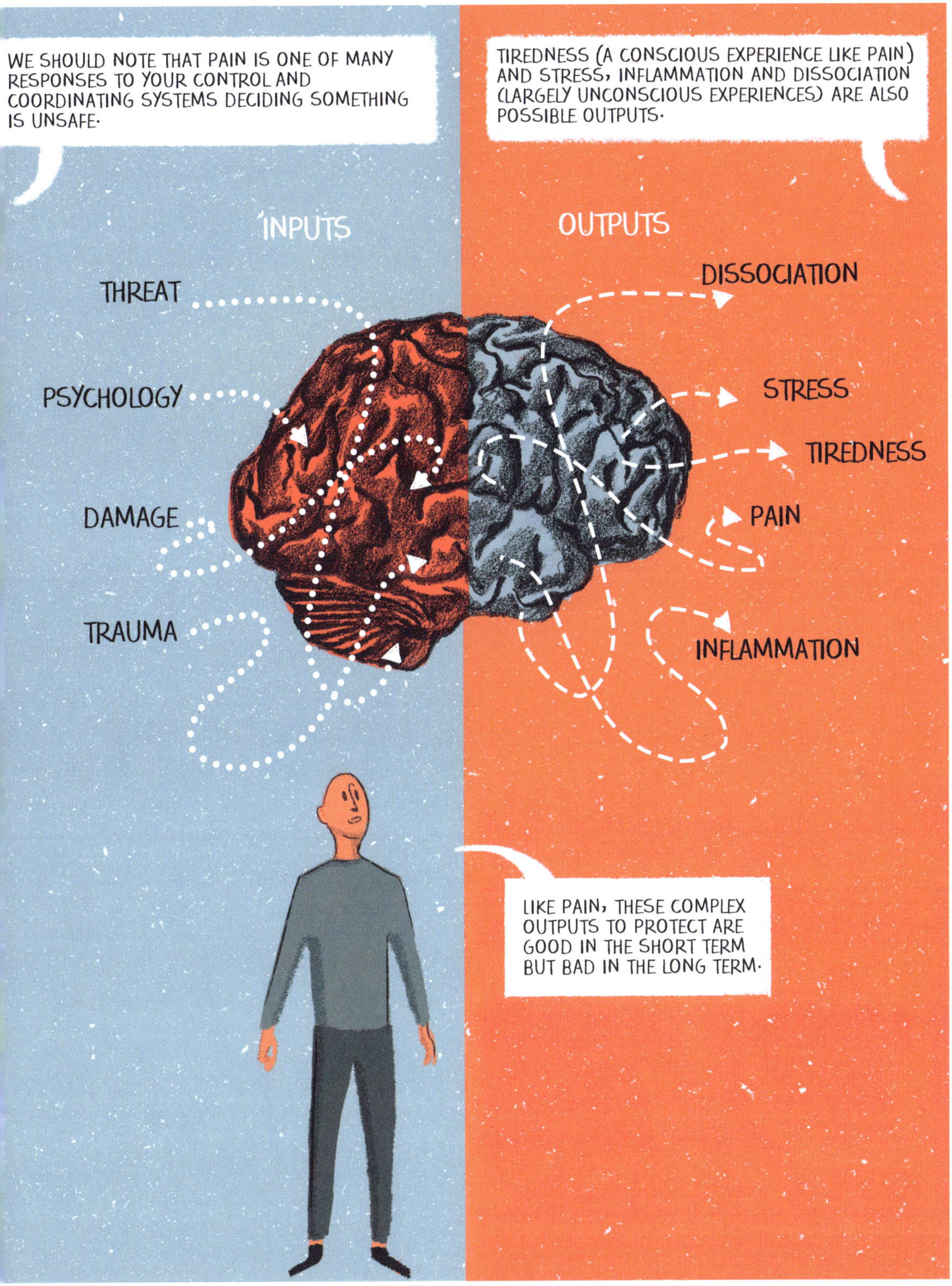

WE SHOULD NOTE THAT PAIN IS ONE OF MANY RESPONSES TO YOUR CONTROL AND COORDINATING SYSTEMS DECIDING SOMETHING IS UNSAFE.
TIREDNESS (A CONSCIOUS EXPERIENCE LIKE PAIN) AND STRESS, INFLAMMATION AND DISSOCIATION (LARGELY UNCONSCIOUS EXPERIENCES) ARE ALSO POSSIBLE OUTPUTS.
INPUTS
OUTPUTS
THREAT
PSYCHOLOGY
DAMAGE
TRAUMA
DISSOCIATION
STRESS
TIREDNESS
PAIN
INFLAMMATION
LIKE PAIN, THESE COMPLEX OUTPUTS TO PROTECT ARE GOOD IN THE SHORT TERM BUT BAD IN THE LONG TERM.

ontrol and coordinating systems' is an attempt to find a phrase that nours intelligence as not just about neurons in the brain. Intelligence is emergent phenomenon generated by trillions of cells communicating oughout the body.

The immune system is increasingly being understood as complex parallel intelligence in the body with memory and learning and a sophisticated range of responses to threat. The immune system is sensitized in chronic inflammation (Thacker et al 2007).

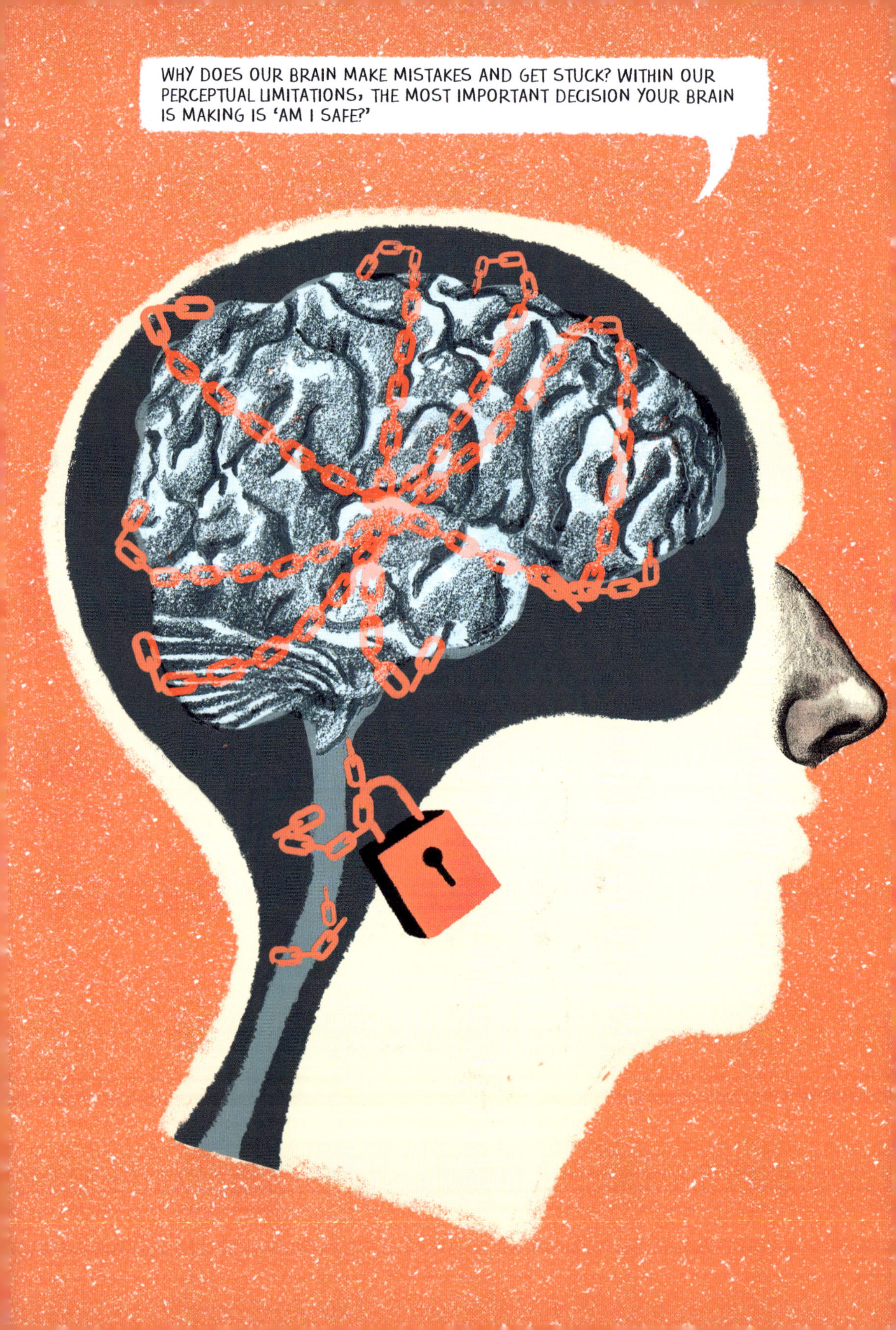
WHY DOES OUR BRAIN MAKE MISTAKES AND GET STUCK? WITHIN OUR PERCEPTUAL LIMITATIONS, THE MOST IMPORTANT DECISION YOUR BRAIN IS MAKING IS 'AM I SAFE?'

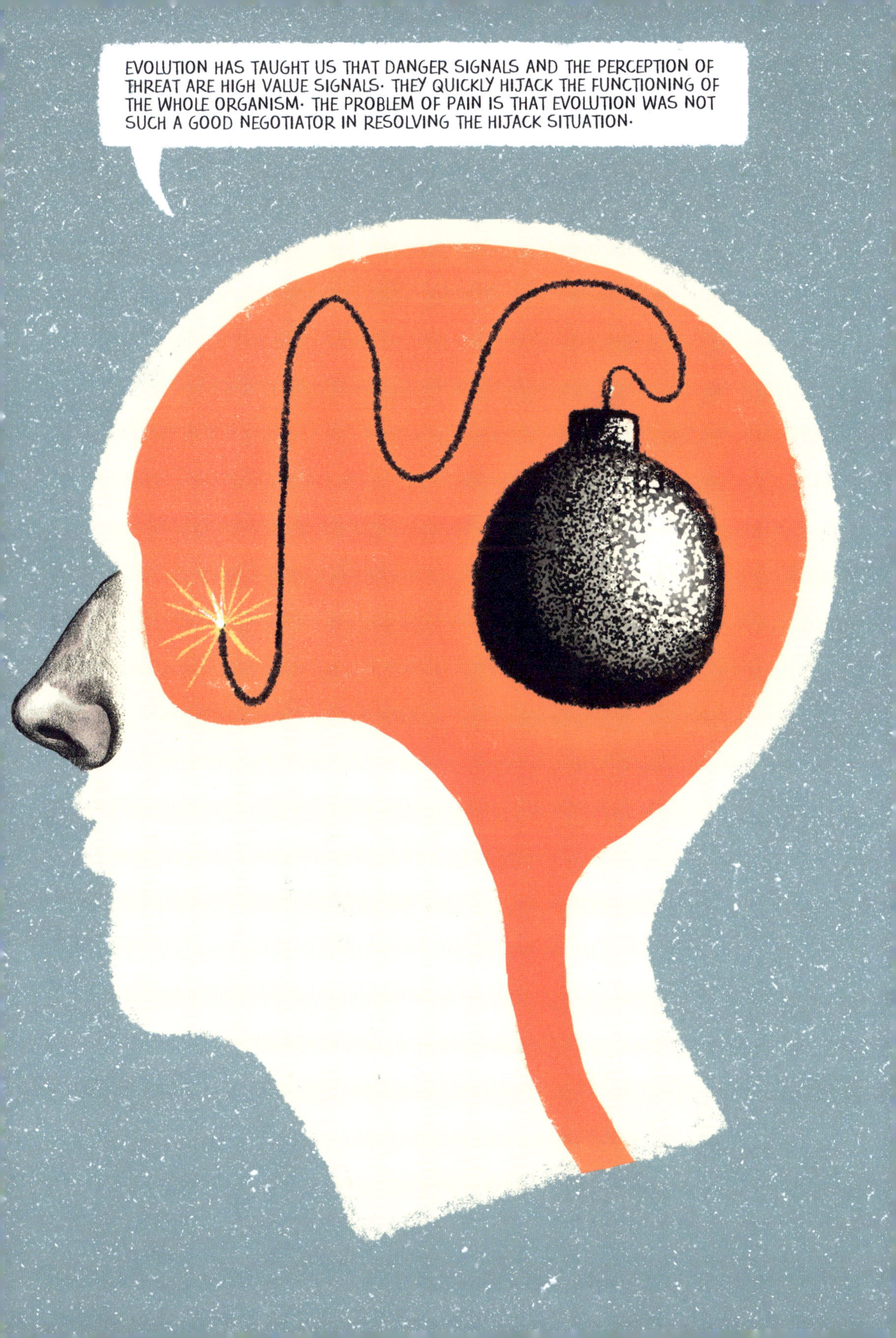
EVOLUTION HAS TAUGHT US THAT DANGER SIGNALS AND THE PERCEPTION OF THREAT ARE HIGH VALUE SIGNALS. THEY QUICKLY HIJACK THE FUNCTIONING OF THE WHOLE ORGANISM. THE PROBLEM OF PAIN IS THAT EVOLUTION WAS NOT SUCH A GOOD NEGOTIATOR IN RESOLVING THE HIJACK SITUATION.

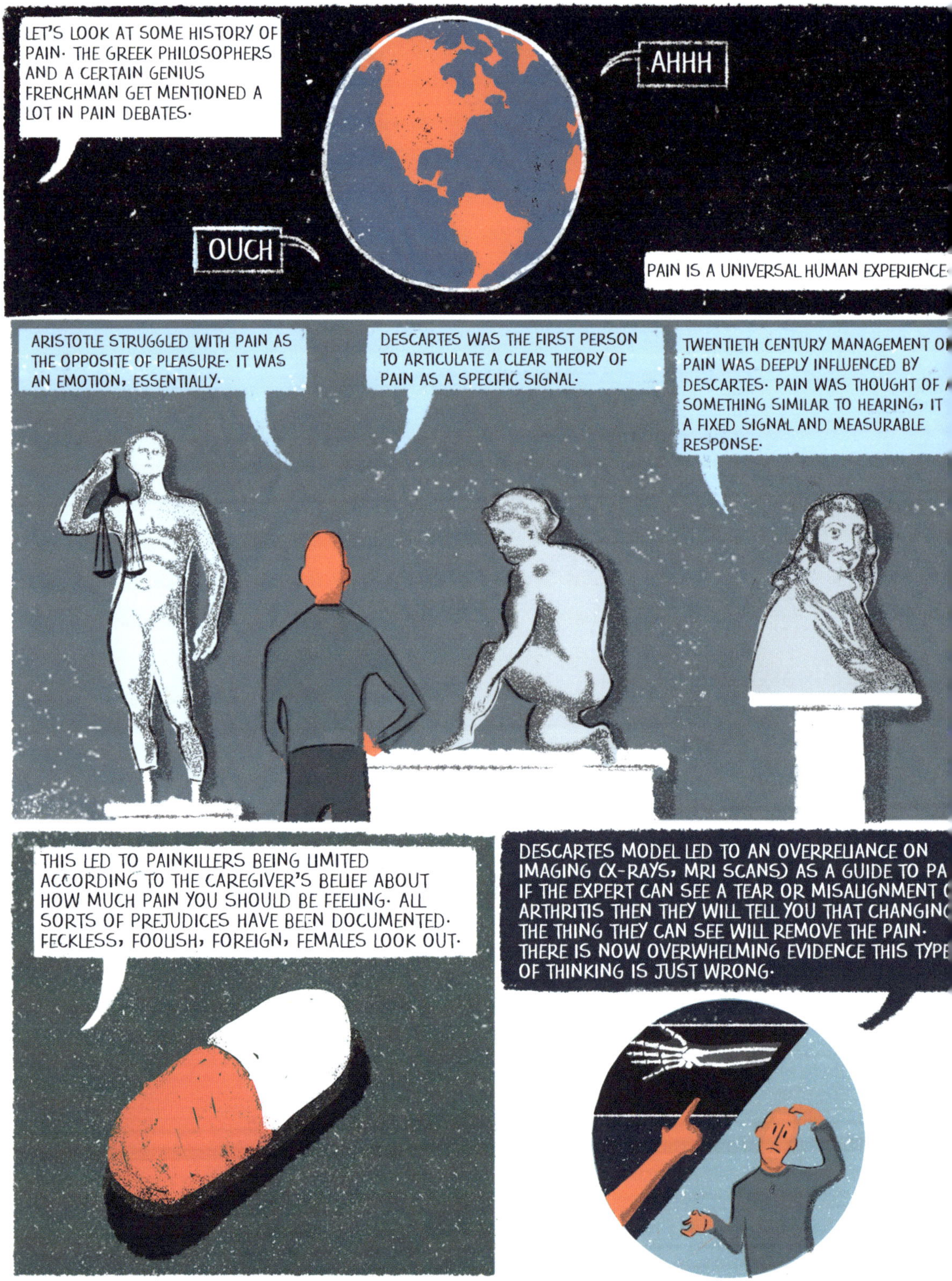

LET'S LOOK AT SOME HISTORY OF PAIN. THE GREEK PHILOSOPHERS AND A CERTAIN GENIUS FRENCHMAN GET MENTIONED A LOT IN PAIN DEBATES.

AHHH

OUCH

PAIN IS A UNIVERSAL HUMAN EXPERIENCE

ARISTOTLE STRUGGLED WITH PAIN AS THE OPPOSITE OF PLEASURE. IT WAS AN EMOTION, ESSENTIALLY.

DESCARTES WAS THE FIRST PERSON TO ARTICULATE A CLEAR THEORY OF PAIN AS A SPECIFIC SIGNAL.

TWENTIETH CENTURY MANAGEMENT OF PAIN WAS DEEPLY INFLUENCED BY DESCARTES. PAIN WAS THOUGHT OF AS SOMETHING SIMILAR TO HEARING, IT A FIXED SIGNAL AND MEASURABLE RESPONSE.

THIS LED TO PAINKILLERS BEING LIMITED ACCORDING TO THE CAREGIVER'S BELIEF ABOUT HOW MUCH PAIN YOU SHOULD BE FEELING. ALL SORTS OF PREJUDICES HAVE BEEN DOCUMENTED. FECKLESS, FOOLISH, FOREIGN, FEMALES LOOK OUT.

DESCARTES MODEL LED TO AN OVERRELIANCE ON IMAGING (X-RAYS, MRI SCANS) AS A GUIDE TO PA IF THE EXPERT CAN SEE A TEAR OR MISALIGNMENT O ARTHRITIS THEN THEY WILL TELL YOU THAT CHANGIN THE THING THEY CAN SEE WILL REMOVE THE PAIN. THERE IS NOW OVERWHELMING EVIDENCE THIS TYPE OF THINKING IS JUST WRONG.

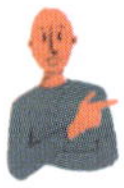

'The evidence that tissue pathology does not explain chronic pain is overwhelming (e.g., in back pain, neck pain, and knee osteoarthritis)' (Moseley 2012a). It is rare for researchers to use the word 'overwhelming'.

Bourke (2014b) is wonderful on how beliefs have affected treatmen She describes a shocking example of young infants, presumably believ to have limited consciousness and memory, having amputations witho anaesthesia as late as the 1970s.

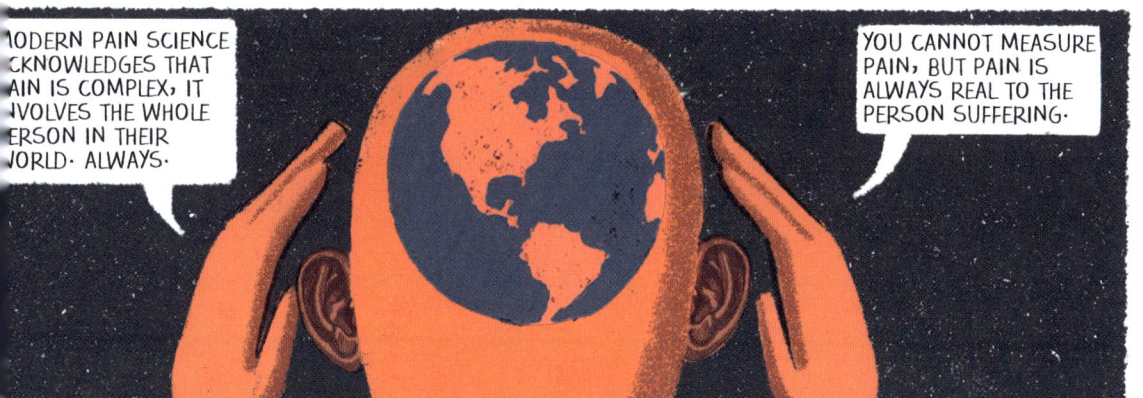

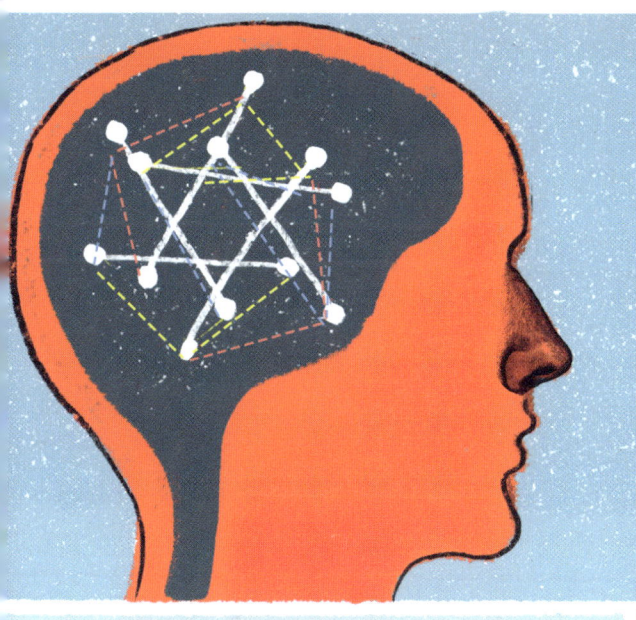

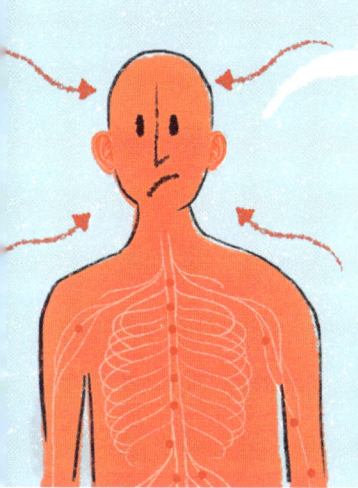

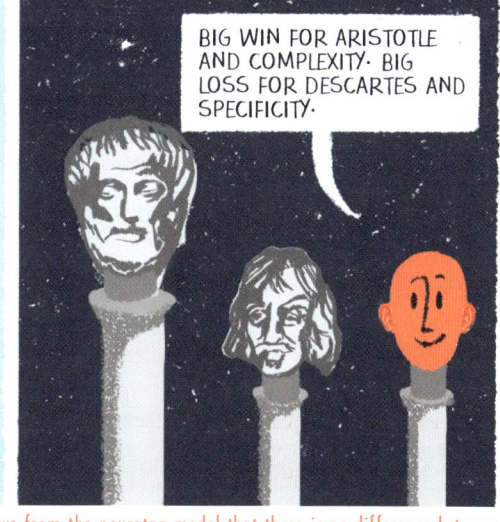

ne claiming to be "in pain" is in pain' (Bourke 2014a). Pain is ve'; it is a 'complex experience that can only be measured by the l reports of patients' (Cervero 2012).

It follows from the neurotag model that there is no difference between emotional pain and physical pain. Similarly, pain and suffering can be used interchangeably, though pain is described by using the body as a reference and suffering is more often expressed as mental angst.

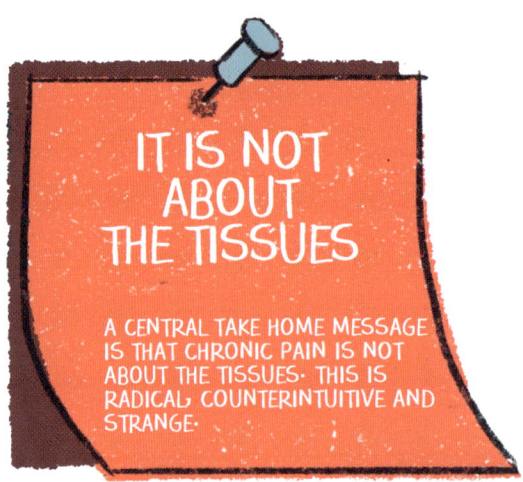
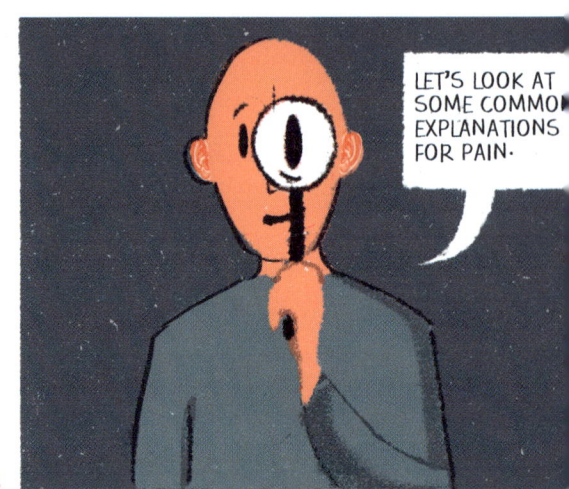
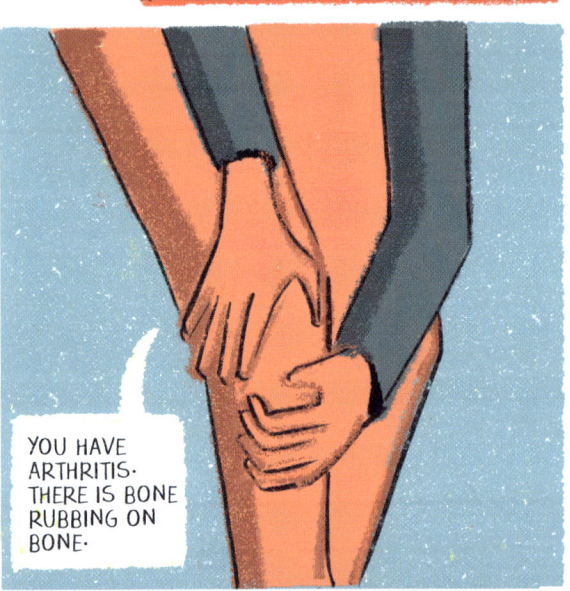
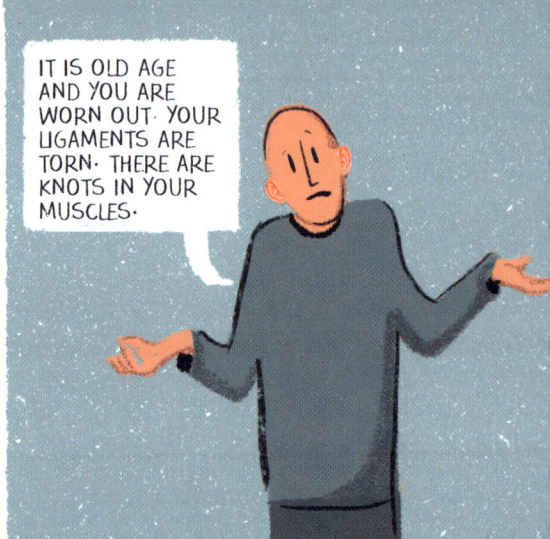
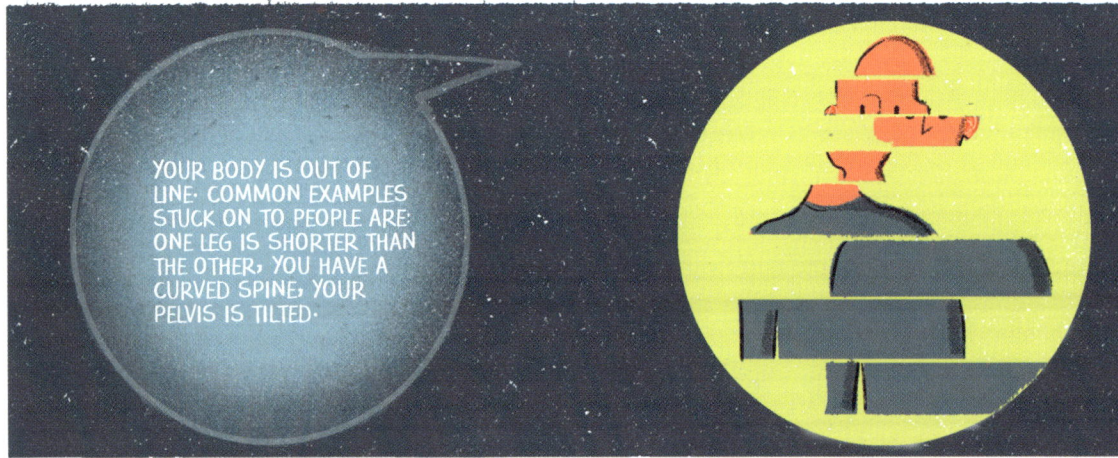

 Getting old is not associated with an increase in back pain. In a large study 'there were no meaningful differences in the frequency of low back pain between younger and older individuals' (Lederman 2010).

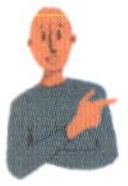

Alignment does not predict back pain. Excessive spinal curves 'failed to show an association with back pain' (Lederman 2010). 'Modern scientific evidence clearly shows that the importance of most bio-"mechanical" problems has been greatly exaggerated' (Ingraham 2014).

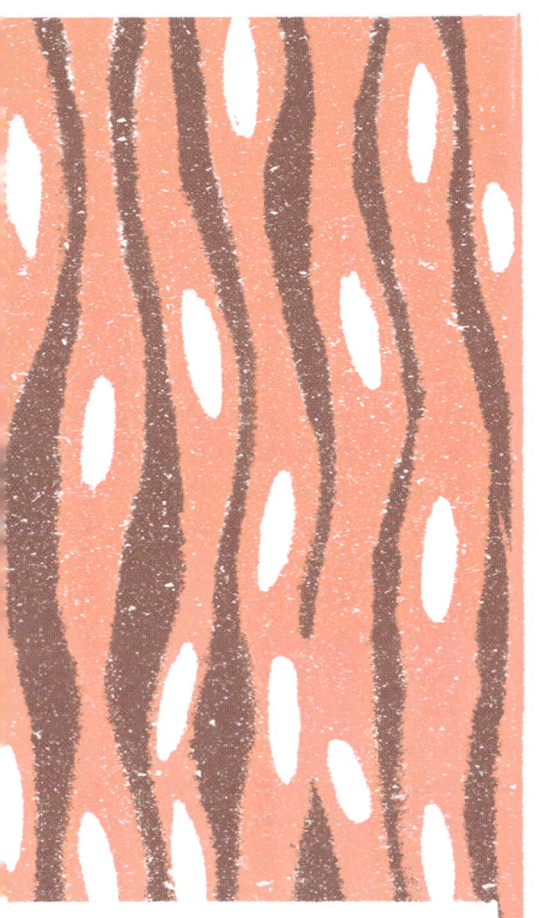

THESE EXPLANATIONS SOUND PLAUSABLE, BUT THERE IS NOW AN OVERWHELMING AMOUNT OF EVIDENCE THAT 'ISSUES IN THE TISSUES' ARE NOT THE CAUSE OF CHRONIC PAIN.

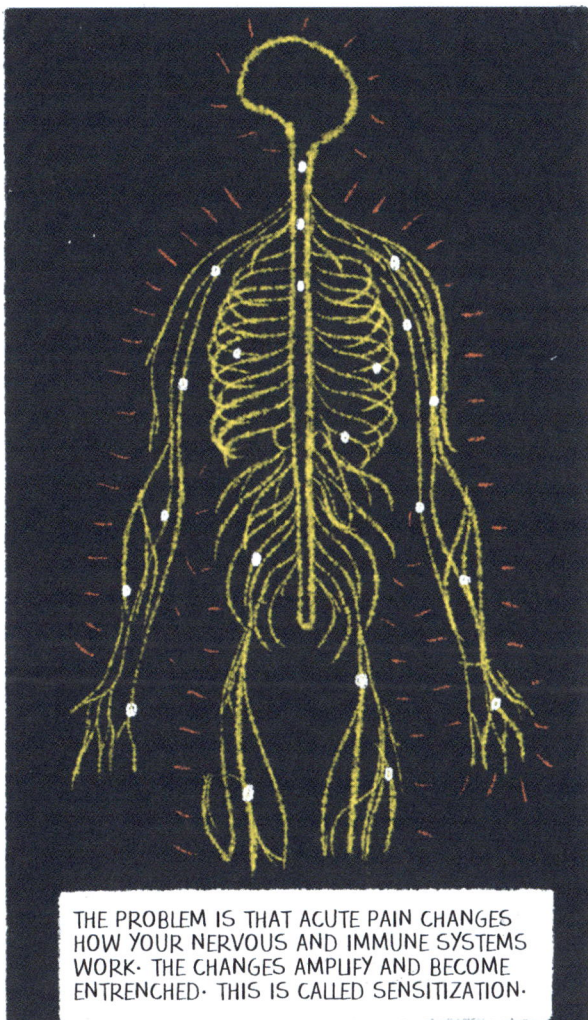

THE PROBLEM IS THAT ACUTE PAIN CHANGES HOW YOUR NERVOUS AND IMMUNE SYSTEMS WORK. THE CHANGES AMPLIFY AND BECOME ENTRENCHED. THIS IS CALLED SENSITIZATION.

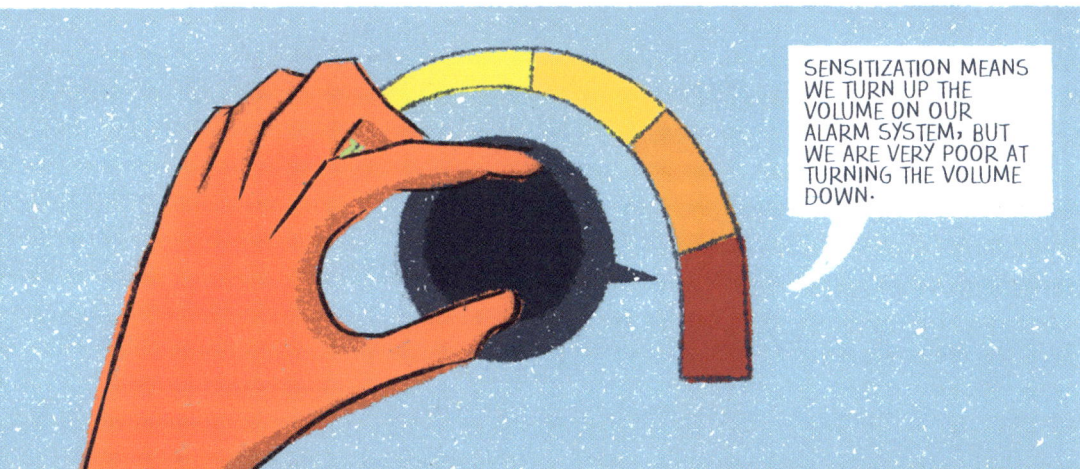

SENSITIZATION MEANS WE TURN UP THE VOLUME ON OUR ALARM SYSTEM, BUT WE ARE VERY POOR AT TURNING THE VOLUME DOWN.

nt pains are often described as grinding.' This word is a 'brain derived struction' used because it 'makes sense mechanically'. '...We all have n out joint surfaces and little bony outgrowths,' '...but most people h worn joints will never know about it' (Butler and Moseley 2003).

Shoulder surgeons, examining the relationship between the severity of rotator cuff (a group of muscles and ligaments in the shoulder) disease and pain, found 'symptoms of pain do not correlate with rotator cuff tear severity' (Dunn et al 2014). Wow, seeing a tear is often used to justify surgery.

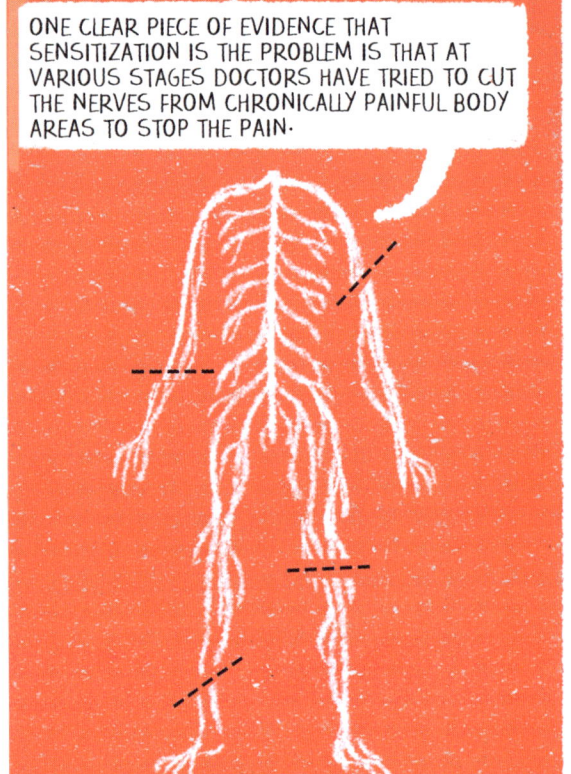

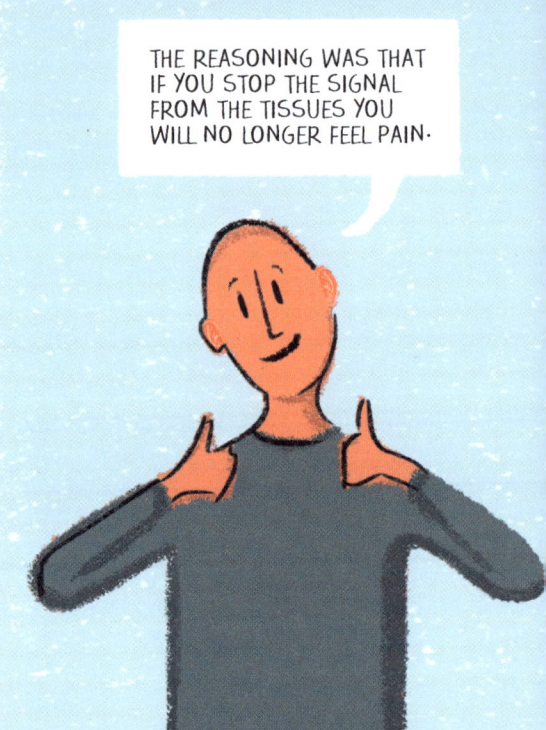

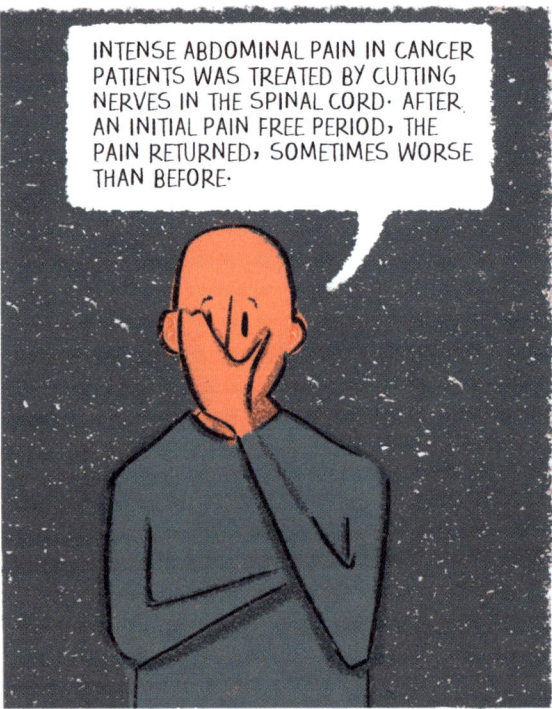

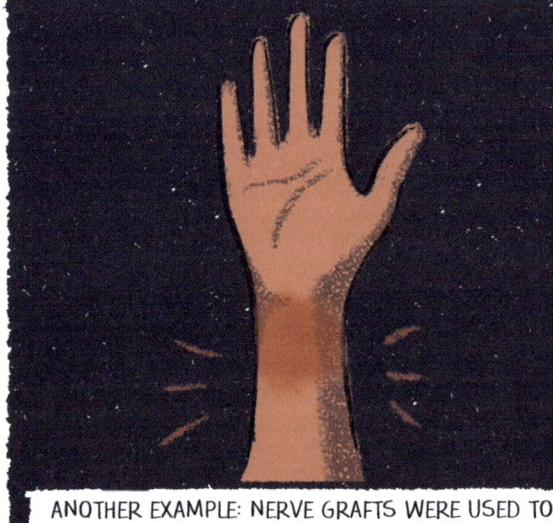

Cervero (2012) describes surgeons in the 1950s cutting bits of the spinal cord to stop severe pain. Initially, on terminal cancer patients, the results were spectacularly good. Patients who lived longer began, tragically, to get pain sensations equal to or worse than the original experience.

Wall (2000) describes wrist surgery to repair median nerves. The pati[ent] had improved hand control but, Wall states, 'angry nerve cells' in the w[rist] had become hyperexcitable and were the cause of the ongoing pain.

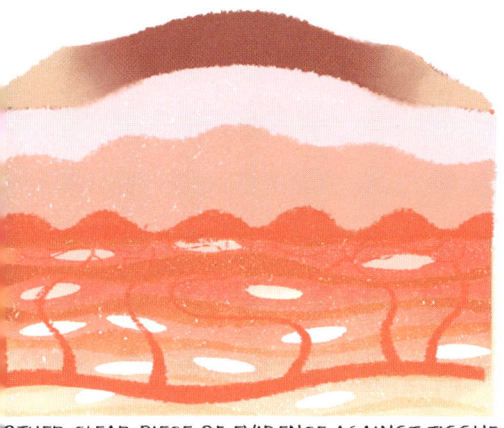

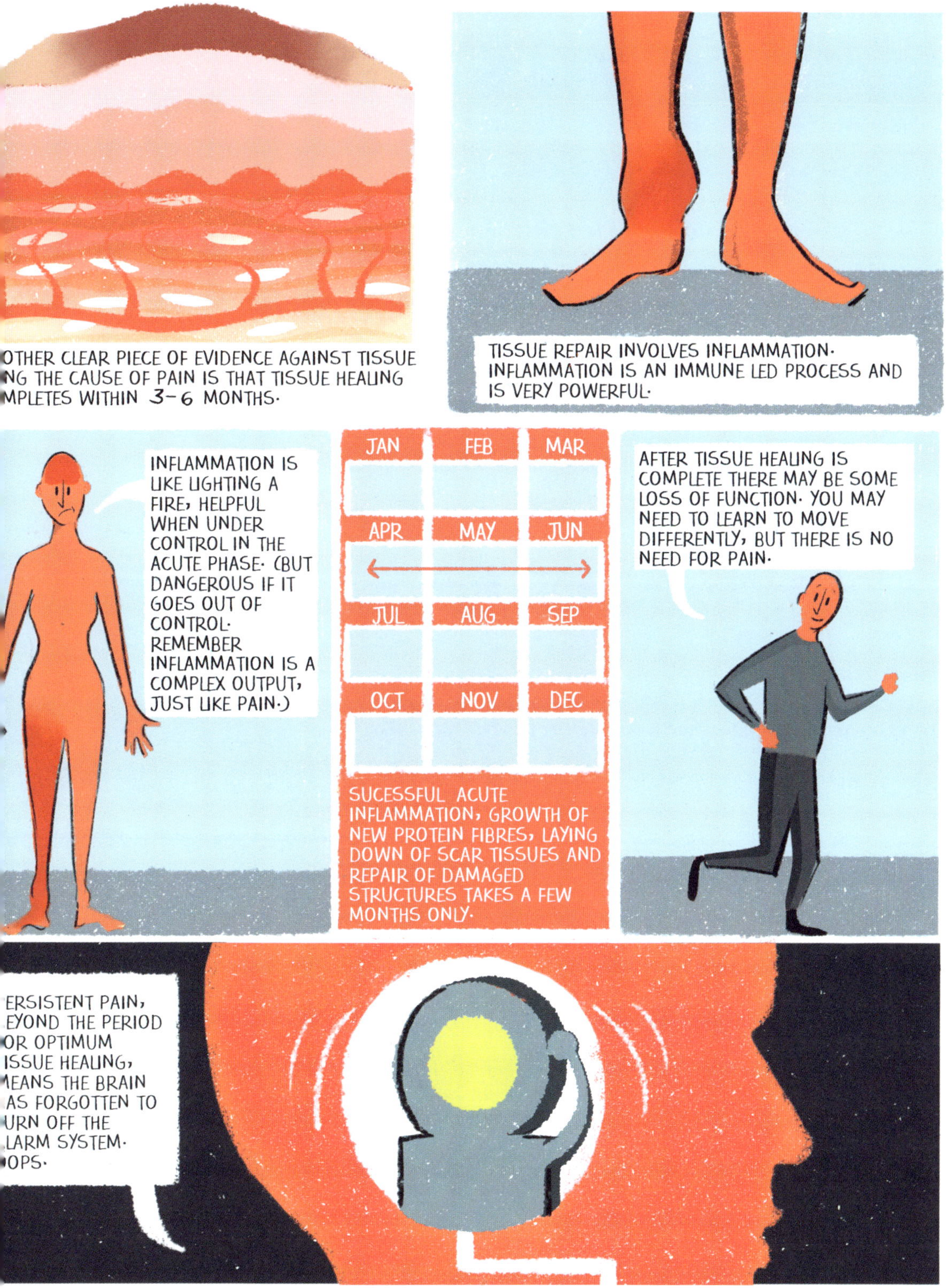

OTHER CLEAR PIECE OF EVIDENCE AGAINST TISSUE [DAMAGE BEI]NG THE CAUSE OF PAIN IS THAT TISSUE HEAL[ING CO]MPLETES WITHIN 3-6 MONTHS.

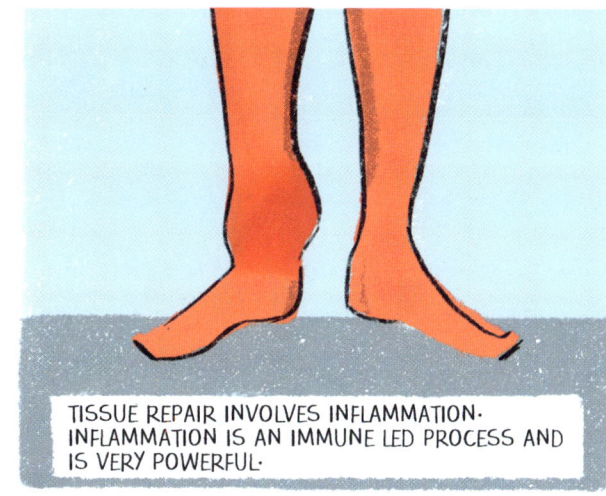

TISSUE REPAIR INVOLVES INFLAMMATION. INFLAMMATION IS AN IMMUNE LED PROCESS AND IS VERY POWERFUL.

INFLAMMATION IS LIKE LIGHTING A FIRE, HELPFUL WHEN UNDER CONTROL IN THE ACUTE PHASE. (BUT DANGEROUS IF IT GOES OUT OF CONTROL. REMEMBER INFLAMMATION IS A COMPLEX OUTPUT, JUST LIKE PAIN.)

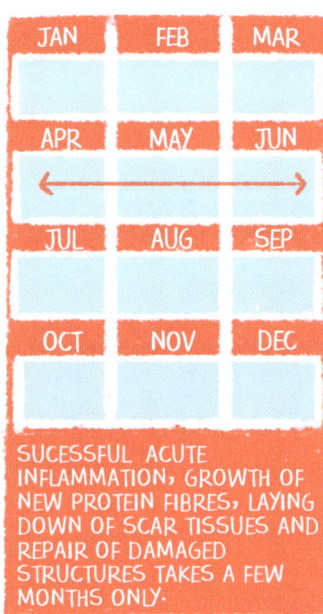

SUCCESSFUL ACUTE INFLAMMATION, GROWTH OF NEW PROTEIN FIBRES, LAYING DOWN OF SCAR TISSUES AND REPAIR OF DAMAGED STRUCTURES TAKES A FEW MONTHS ONLY.

AFTER TISSUE HEALING IS COMPLETE THERE MAY BE SOME LOSS OF FUNCTION. YOU MAY NEED TO LEARN TO MOVE DIFFERENTLY, BUT THERE IS NO NEED FOR PAIN.

[P]ERSISTENT PAIN, [B]EYOND THE PERIOD [F]OR OPTIMUM [T]ISSUE HEALING, [M]EANS THE BRAIN [H]AS FORGOTTEN TO [T]URN OFF THE [A]LARM SYSTEM. [O]OPS.

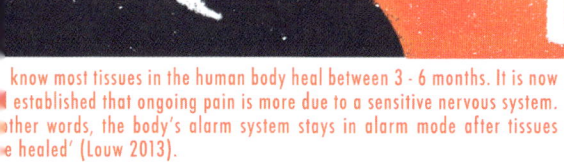

'[We] know most tissues in the human body heal between 3 - 6 months. It is now [well] established that ongoing pain is more due to a sensitive nervous system. [In o]ther words, the body's alarm system stays in alarm mode after tissues [ar]e healed' (Louw 2013).

Medicine 'assumes that injury and pain are the same issue; therefore, an increase in pain means increased tissue injury and increased tissue issues lead to more pain. This model (called the Cartesian model of pain) is over 350 years old, and it's incorrect' (Louw 2014).

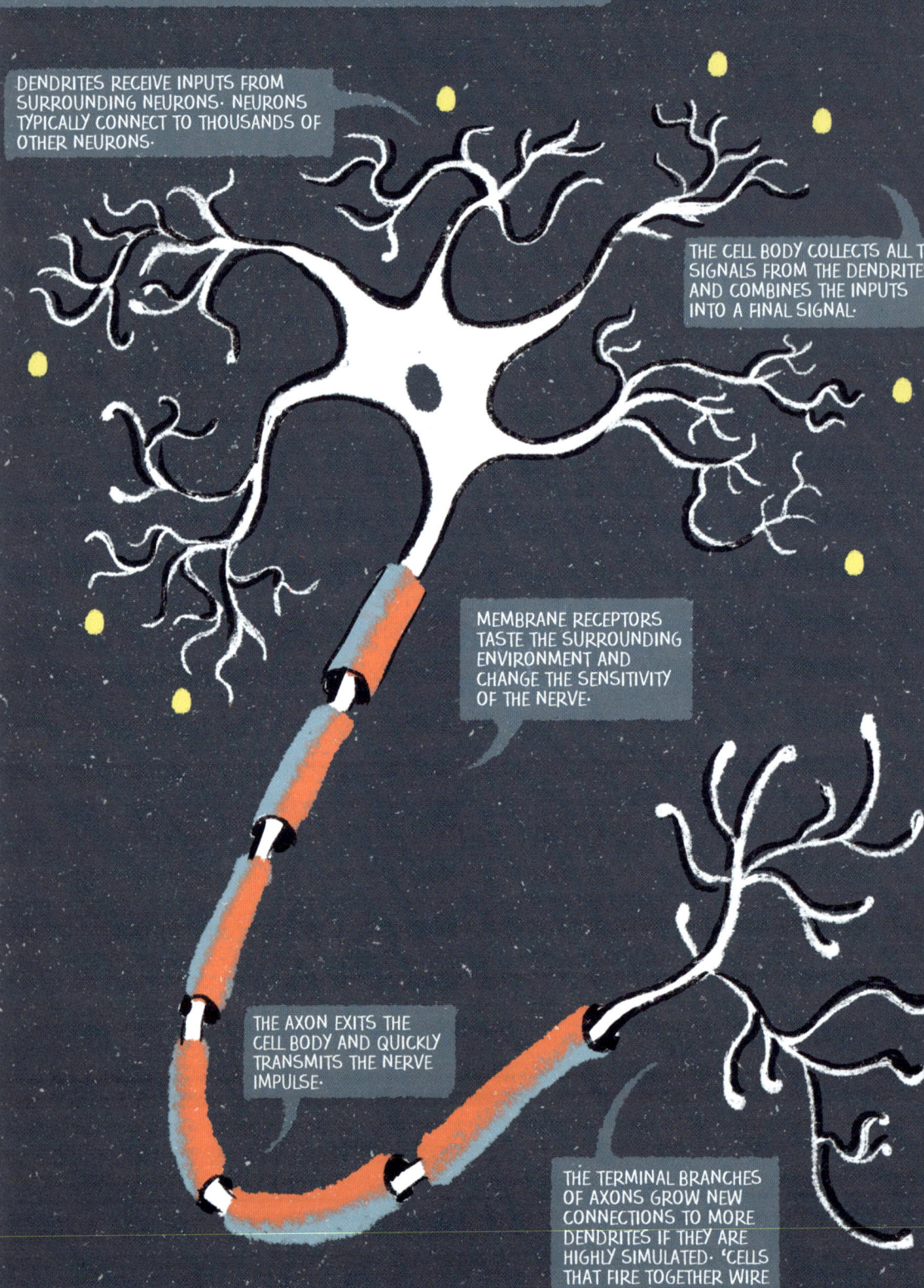

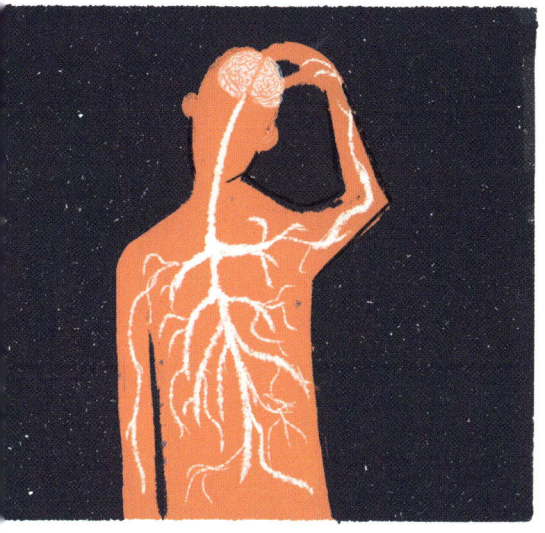

NERVES ARE MUCH MORE COMPLEX THAN YOU PROBABLY REALIZE. A SIMPLE ELECTRIC CABLE OR SIMPLE SWITCH IS AN OVERSIMPLIFICATION.

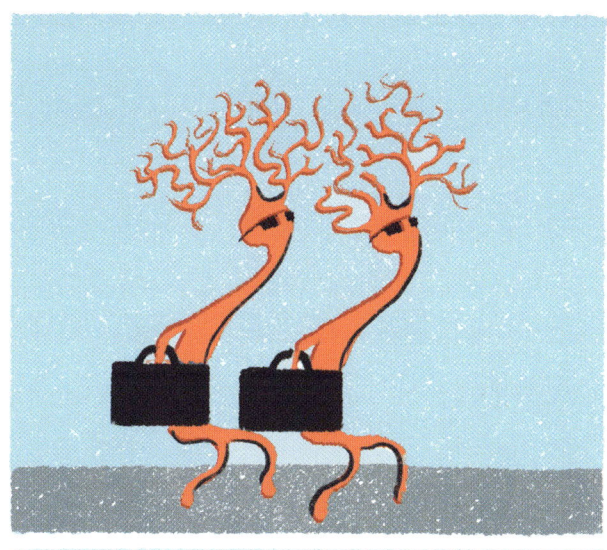

NERVE CELLS ARE LITTLE AGENTS WITH THEIR OWN AGENDA. THEY ADAPT TO THE DEMANDS PLACED ON THEM.

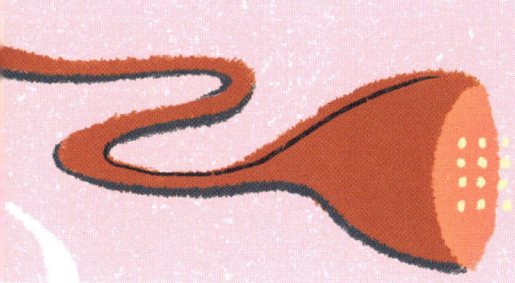

[NE]URONS CONNECT VIA SYNAPSES. AT THE SYNAPSE, [A] WAVE OF ELECTRIC CHARGE ALONG THE AXON [CA]USES CHEMICALS CALLED NEUROTRANSMITTERS TO [BE] RELEASED.

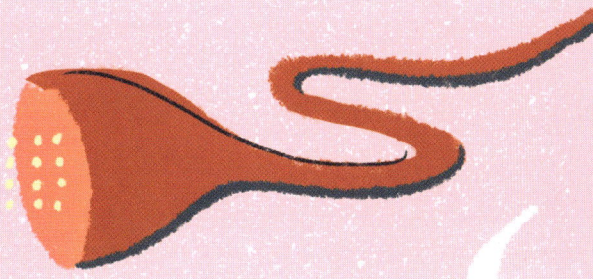

ON THE OTHER SIDE OF THE SYNAPSE ANOTHER CELL (USUALLY ANOTHER NEURON) ABSORBS THE NEUROTRANSMITTERS VIA MEMBRANE RECEPTORS.

[T]HE SCIENCE OF NEUROTRANSMITTERS AND [M]EMBRANE RECEPTORS IS WONDERFULLY COMPLEX, [B]UT IS VERY IMPORTANT IN UNDERSTANDING HOW [BR]AIN WORKS.

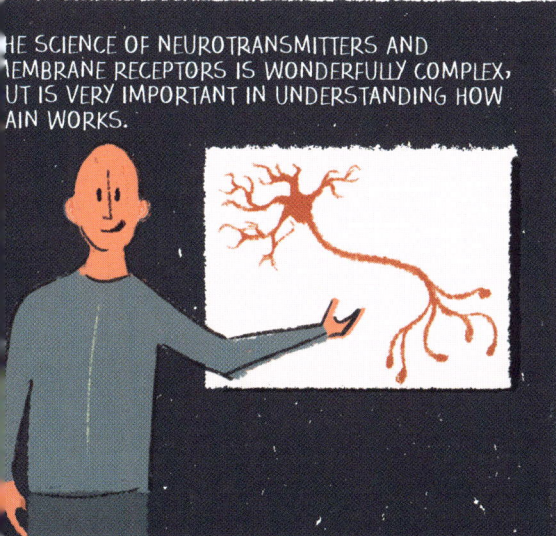

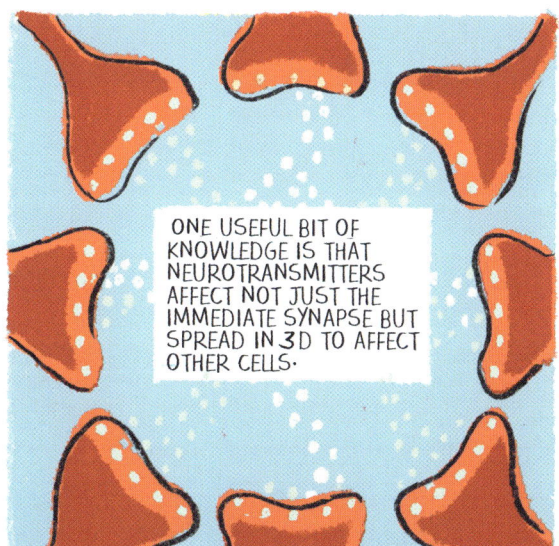

ONE USEFUL BIT OF KNOWLEDGE IS THAT NEUROTRANSMITTERS AFFECT NOT JUST THE IMMEDIATE SYNAPSE BUT SPREAD IN 3D TO AFFECT OTHER CELLS.

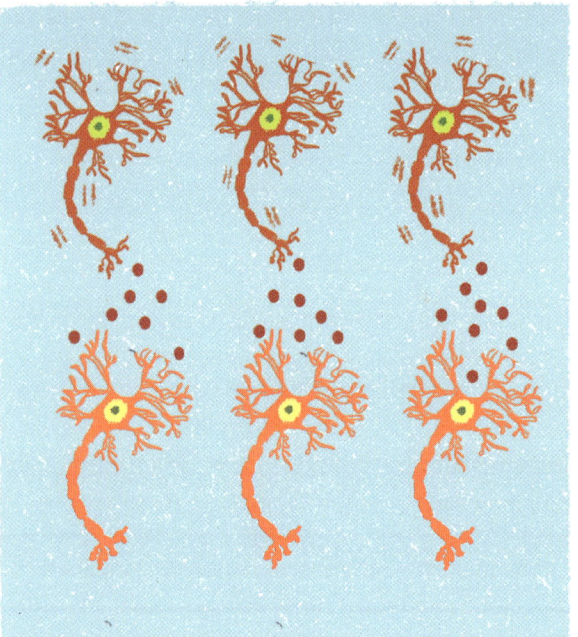

DANGER SIGNALS ARE BAD NEWS THAT TRAVELS FAST. THE ASSOCIATED NEUROTRANSMITTERS QUICKLY AFFECT OTHER CELLS. ANGRY NEURONS SHOUT A LOT.

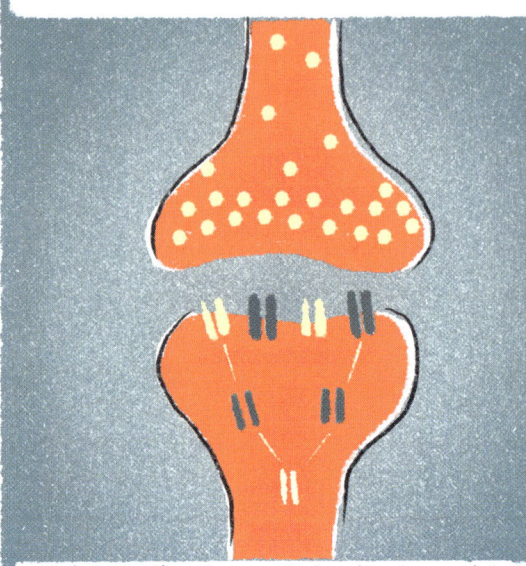

ANOTHER USEFUL BIT OF INFORMATION IS THAT MEMBRANE RECEPTORS CHANGE ALL THE TIME. NEW RECEPTORS ARE INSERTED INTO THE CELL WALL.

THEY QUICKLY SENSITIZE NEURONS TO CIRCULATING STRESS HORMONES, INFLAMMATORY SIGNALS AND DANGER NEUROTRANSMITTERS.

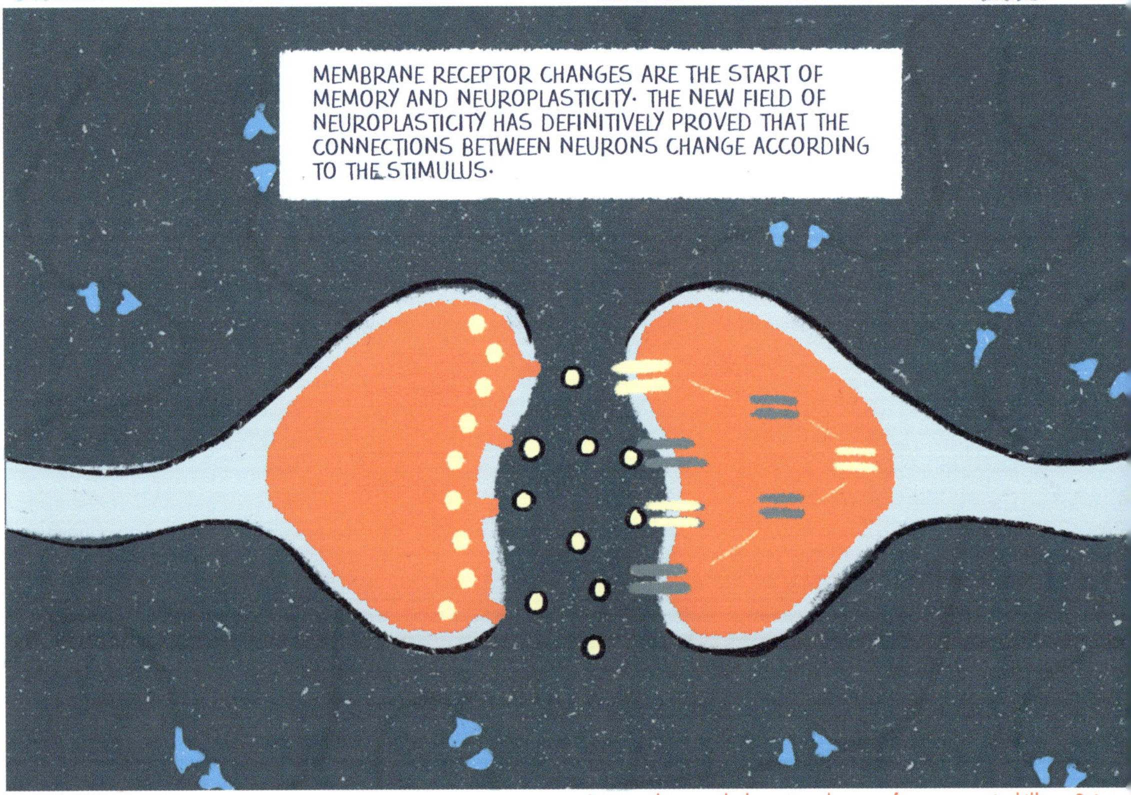

MEMBRANE RECEPTOR CHANGES ARE THE START OF MEMORY AND NEUROPLASTICITY. THE NEW FIELD OF NEUROPLASTICITY HAS DEFINITIVELY PROVED THAT THE CONNECTIONS BETWEEN NEURONS CHANGE ACCORDING TO THE STIMULUS.

Membrane receptors and the activity in synapses are often the targets of pain killing drugs. Anaesthetics have transformed surgery. Common pain killers are very useful drugs.

It is good to regularly review the use of stronger pain killers. Opiates have difficult side effects, generate addiction, sensitize the nervous sys and tolerance means you will need more. Check YouTube: 'Brainman stop opiod'.

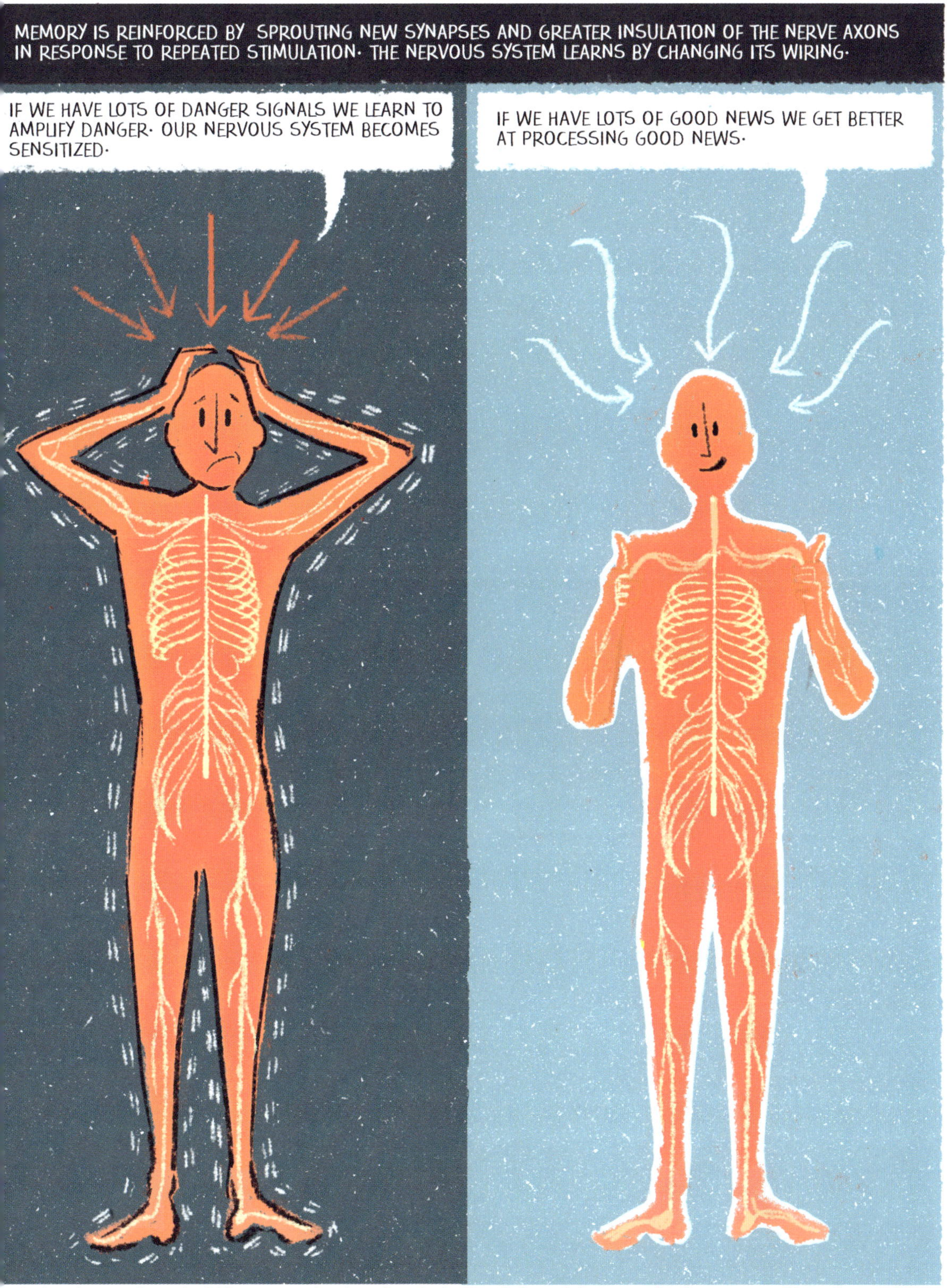

MEMORY IS REINFORCED BY SPROUTING NEW SYNAPSES AND GREATER INSULATION OF THE NERVE AXONS IN RESPONSE TO REPEATED STIMULATION. THE NERVOUS SYSTEM LEARNS BY CHANGING ITS WIRING.

IF WE HAVE LOTS OF DANGER SIGNALS WE LEARN TO AMPLIFY DANGER. OUR NERVOUS SYSTEM BECOMES SENSITIZED.

IF WE HAVE LOTS OF GOOD NEWS WE GET BETTER AT PROCESSING GOOD NEWS.

velo (2012) states that end of life pain can cheaply and easily be ieved with improved availability of existing drugs; world wide lack of ess to effective pain relief is a political problem leading to needless fering.

Bourke (2014a) documents a lot of unnecessary suffering due to inefficient administration of stronger prescription pain killers.

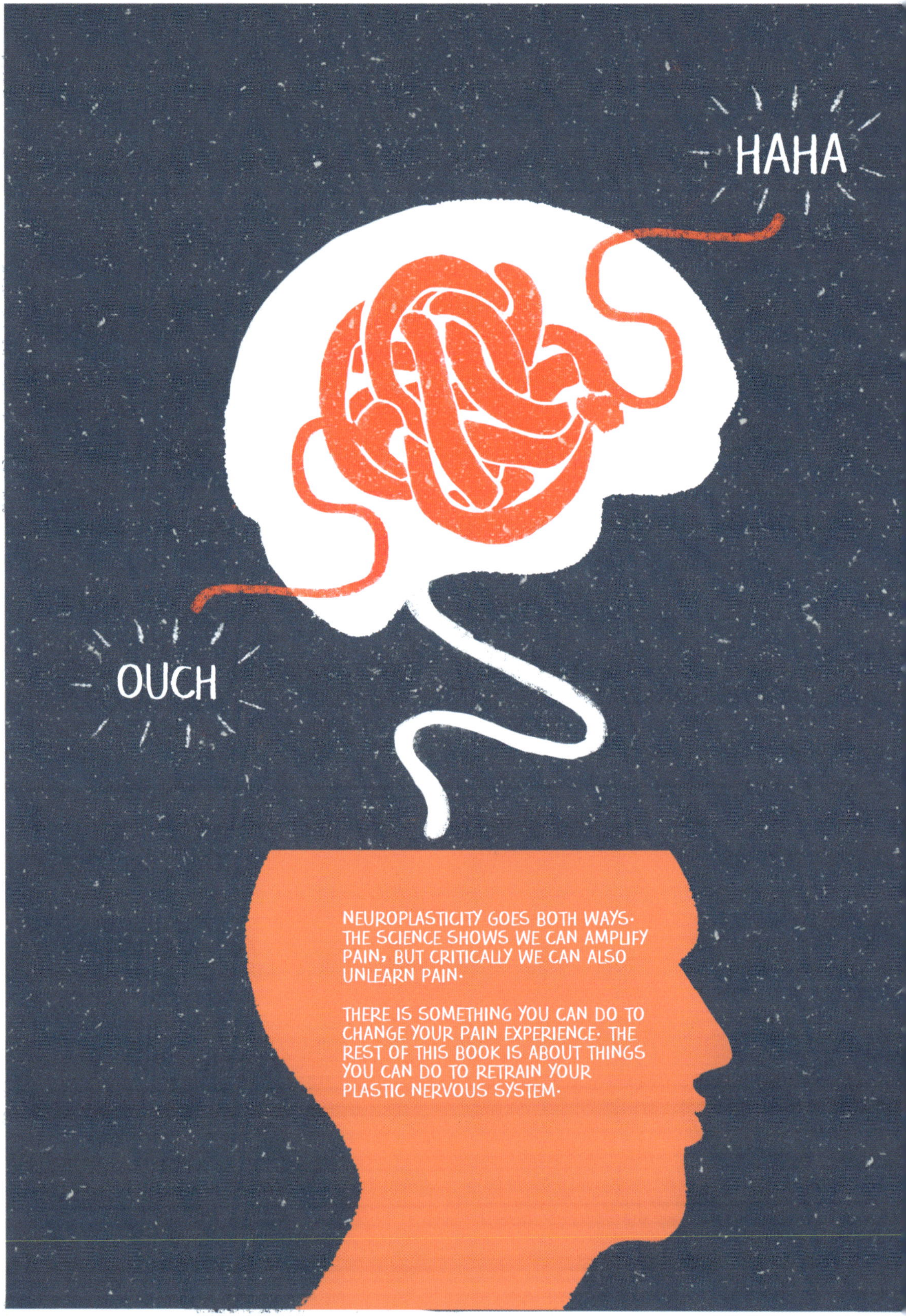
HAHA
OUCH
NEUROPLASTICITY GOES BOTH WAYS. THE SCIENCE SHOWS WE CAN AMPLIFY PAIN, BUT CRITICALLY WE CAN ALSO UNLEARN PAIN.
THERE IS SOMETHING YOU CAN DO TO CHANGE YOUR PAIN EXPERIENCE. THE REST OF THIS BOOK IS ABOUT THINGS YOU CAN DO TO RETRAIN YOUR PLASTIC NERVOUS SYSTEM.

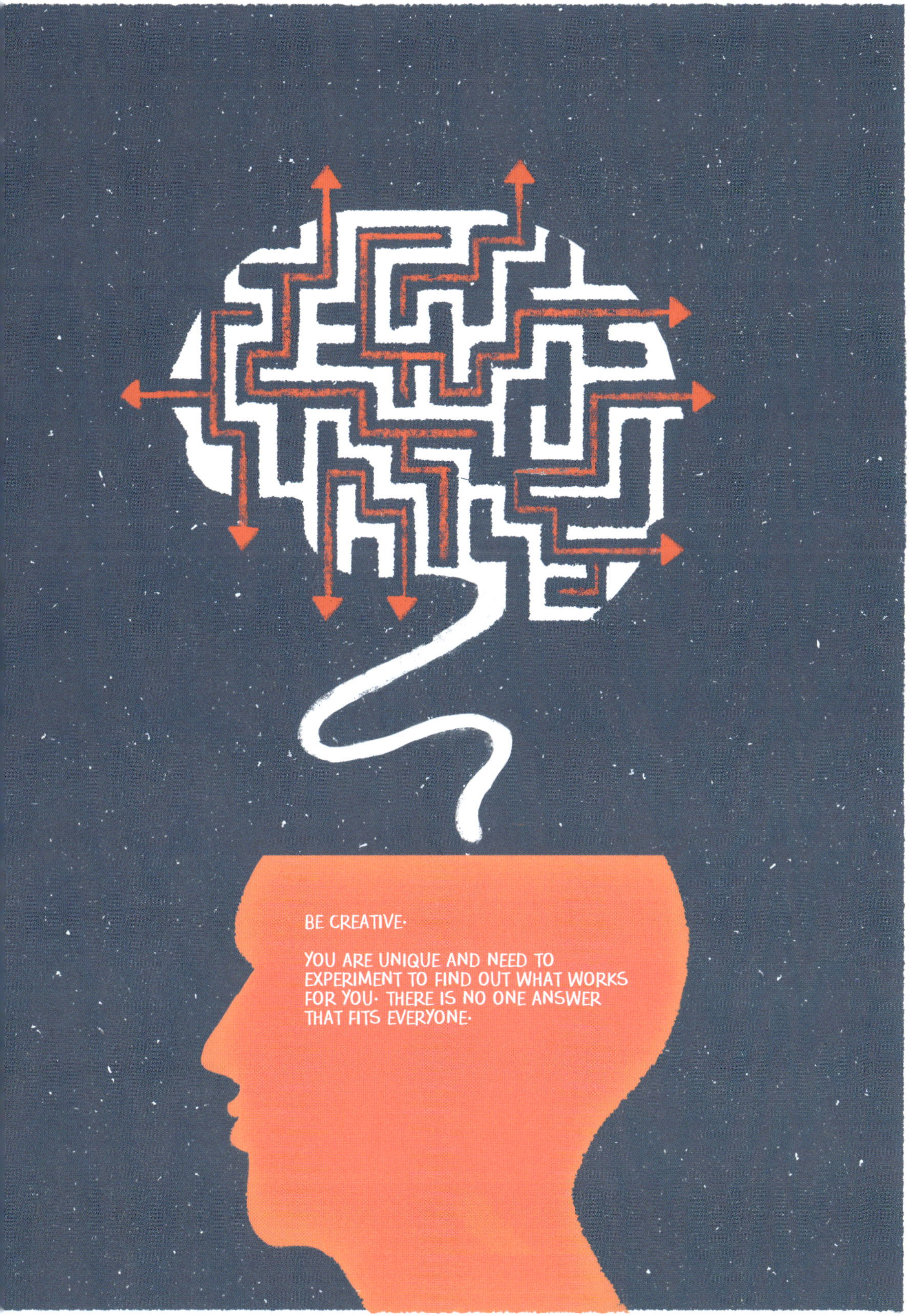
BE CREATIVE.
YOU ARE UNIQUE AND NEED TO EXPERIMENT TO FIND OUT WHAT WORKS FOR YOU. THERE IS NO ONE ANSWER THAT FITS EVERYONE.

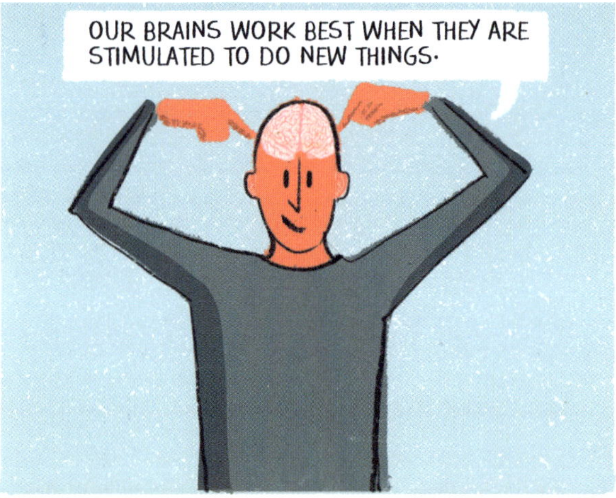
OUR BRAINS WORK BEST WHEN THEY ARE STIMULATED TO DO NEW THINGS.

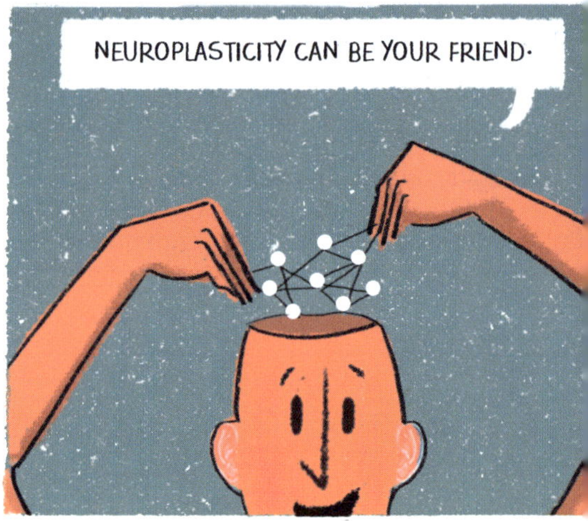
NEUROPLASTICITY CAN BE YOUR FRIEND.

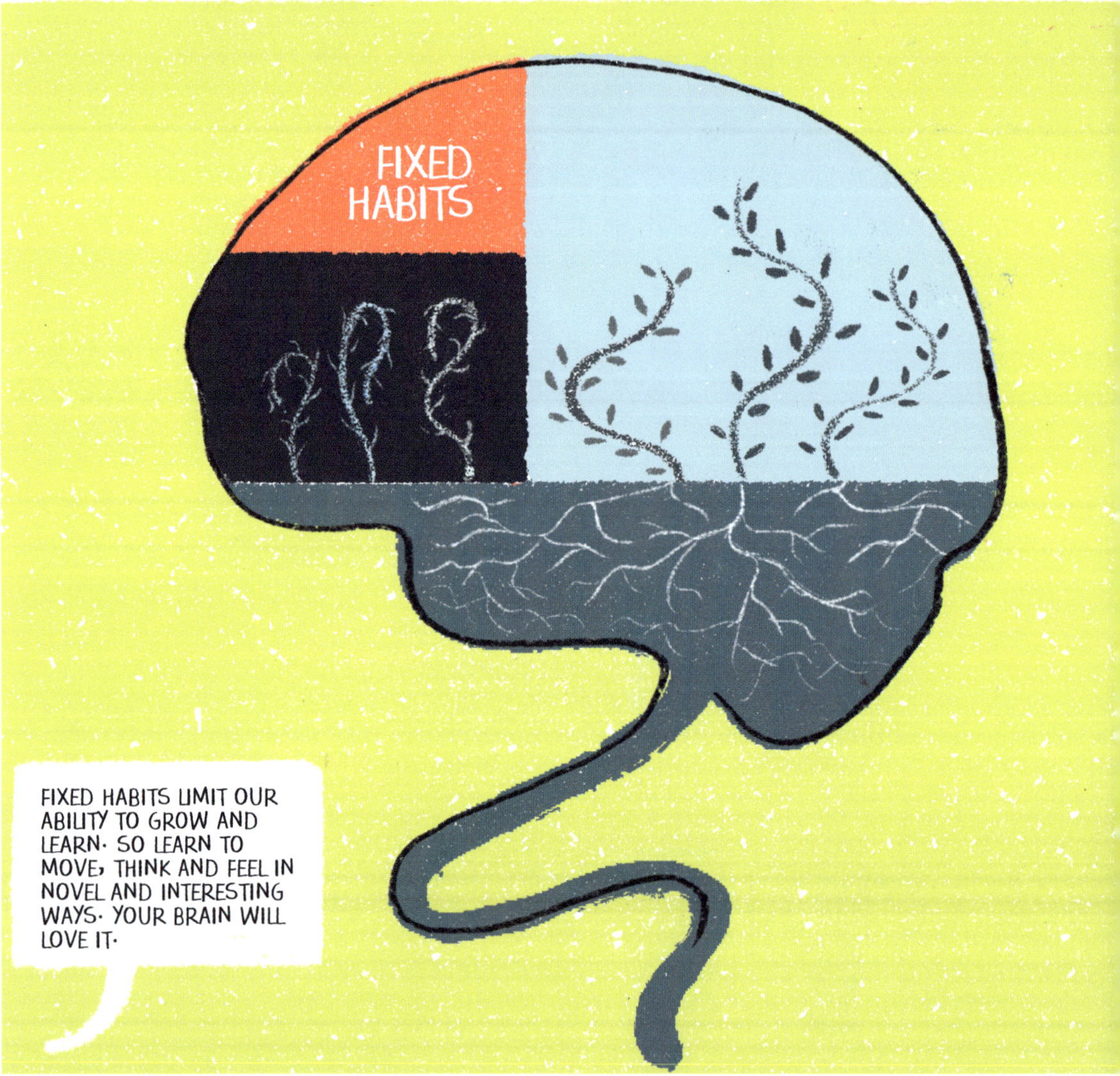
FIXED HABITS
FIXED HABITS LIMIT OUR ABILITY TO GROW AND LEARN. SO LEARN TO MOVE, THINK AND FEEL IN NOVEL AND INTERESTING WAYS. YOUR BRAIN WILL LOVE IT.

'Stereotyping is the enemy - exercise the brain with a variety of movement, action and challenge' (Merzenich 2013).

Michael Merzenich is a huge figure in the science of neuroplasticity. H very optimistic about our ability to enhance the functioning of our 'sc wired' nervous system.

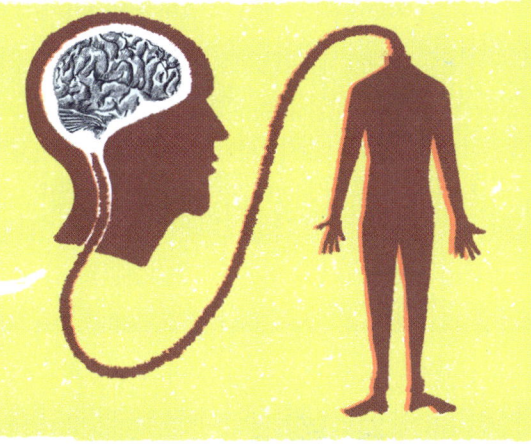

BRAINS NEED TO BE REMINDED OF THE REAL BODY ALL THE TIME. THE BODY NEUROTAG NEEDS CONSTANT FEEDING OR OUR "VIRTUAL BODY" BECOMES MORE ABSTRACT.

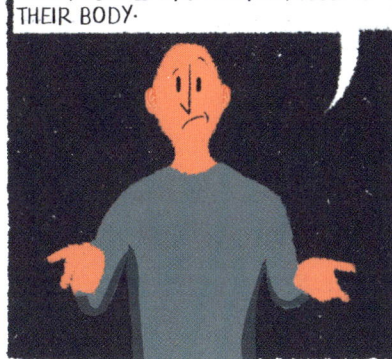

ONE OF THE BIGGEST INSIGHTS I HAVE HAD FROM CLINICAL EXPERIENCE IS MOST PEOPLE ARE POOR AT FEELING THEIR BODY.

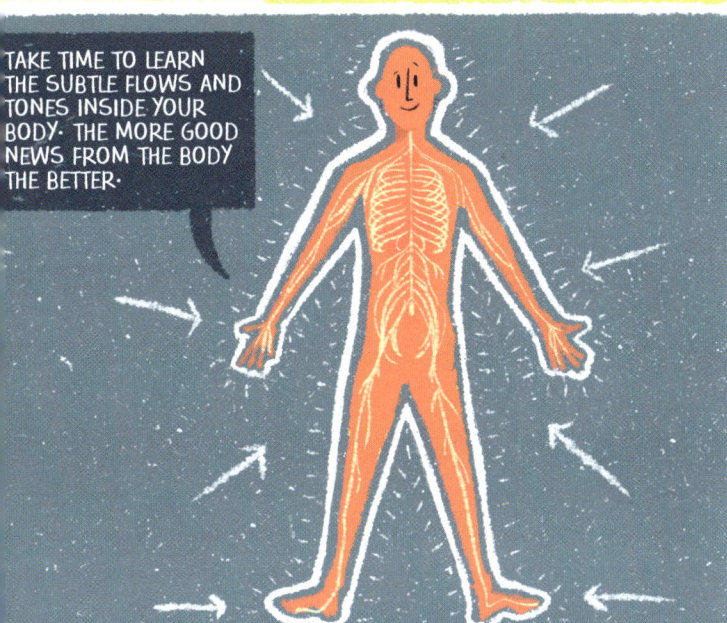

TAKE TIME TO LEARN THE SUBTLE FLOWS AND TONES INSIDE YOUR BODY. THE MORE GOOD NEWS FROM THE BODY THE BETTER.

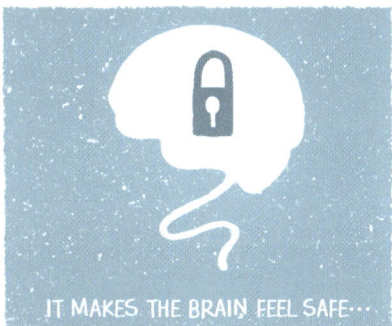

IT MAKES THE BRAIN FEEL SAFE...

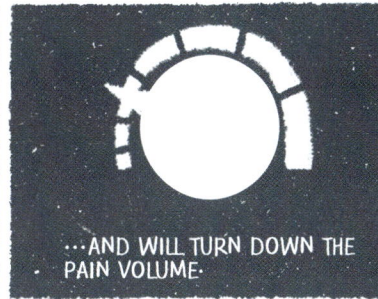

...AND WILL TURN DOWN THE PAIN VOLUME.

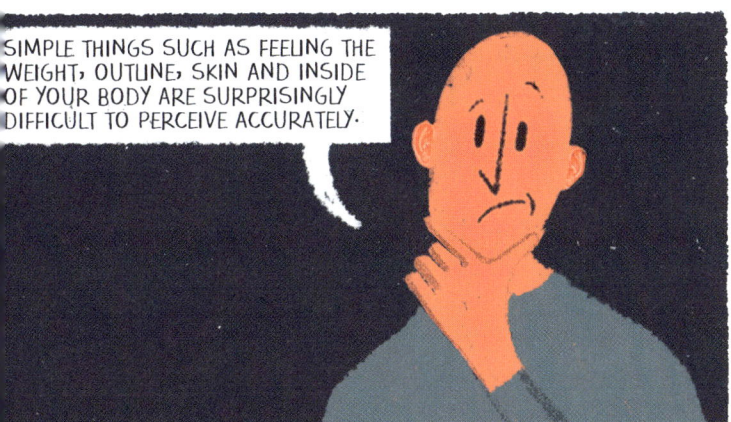

SIMPLE THINGS SUCH AS FEELING THE WEIGHT, OUTLINE, SKIN AND INSIDE OF YOUR BODY ARE SURPRISINGLY DIFFICULT TO PERCEIVE ACCURATELY.

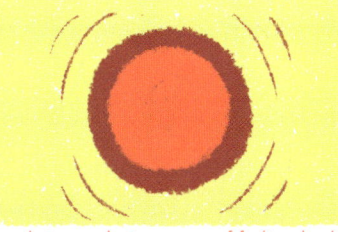

IT IS USEFUL TO REDUCE THE SENSATION YOU EXPERIENCE TO REALLY SIMPLE DESCRIPTIVE WORDS. IS IT HOT OR COLD, MOVING OR FIXED, QUICK OR SLOW, BIG OR SMALL? PAIN MAY BECOME A 'WARM, PULSING AREA THE SIZE OF A PLUM'.

'We don't need a body to feel a body.' This is the amazing conclusion of pain pioneer Ronald Melzack (Melzack and Katz 2013). Treatments that use skillful touch can really help you find your body.

There is lots of evidence accumulating on the importance of feeling the slow background tone of your body (interoception) as well as joints and muscles (proprioception). It takes practice to sense your organs and the internal feel of your limbs, but doing so will pay you back in dividends.

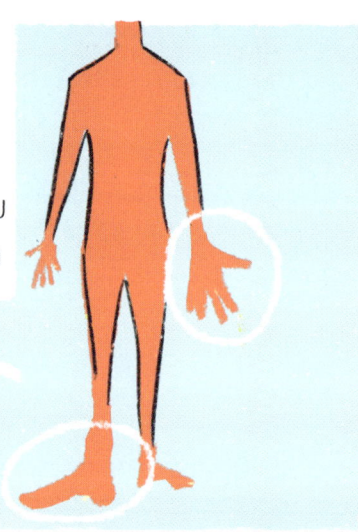
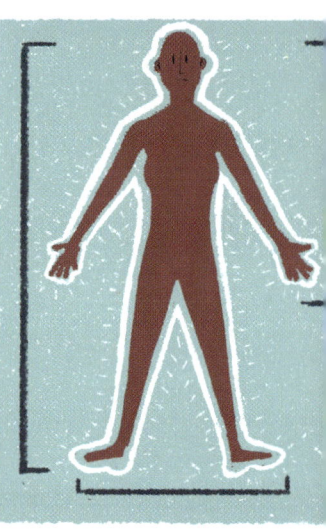
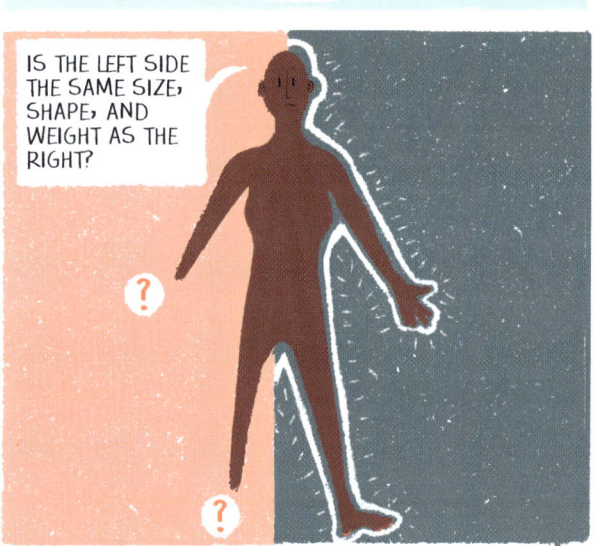
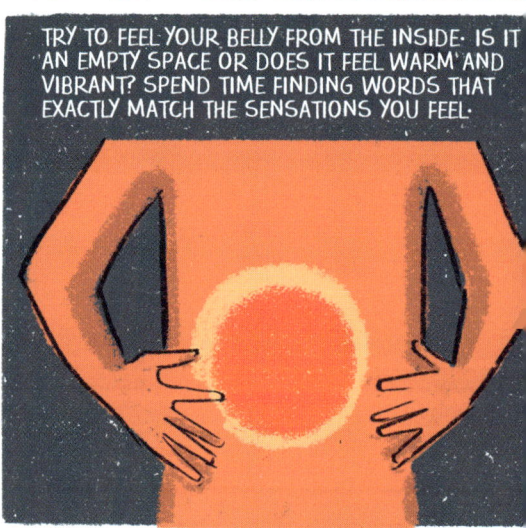
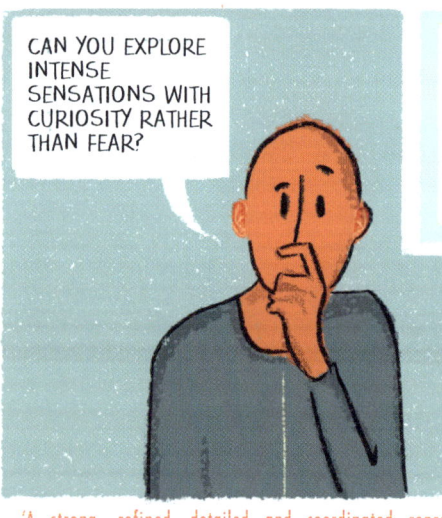
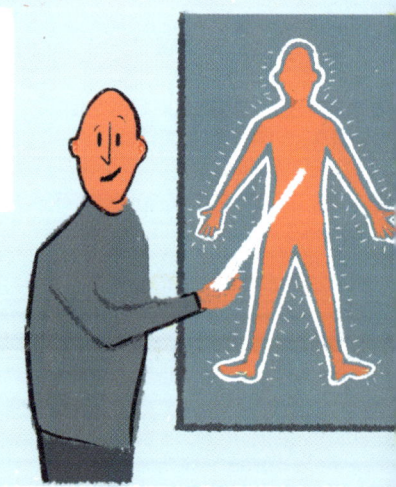

'A strong, refined, detailed and coordinated representation of information from any given region of your body is, by its fundamental nature, anti-pain' (Merzenich 2013).

The Mindfulness-Based Stress Reduction model is an accessible, researche[d] and secular meditation method (Kabat-Zinn 2013). Zen Mind Beginner's Mi[nd] (Suzuki 1970) is an enduring classic on doing less and achieving more.

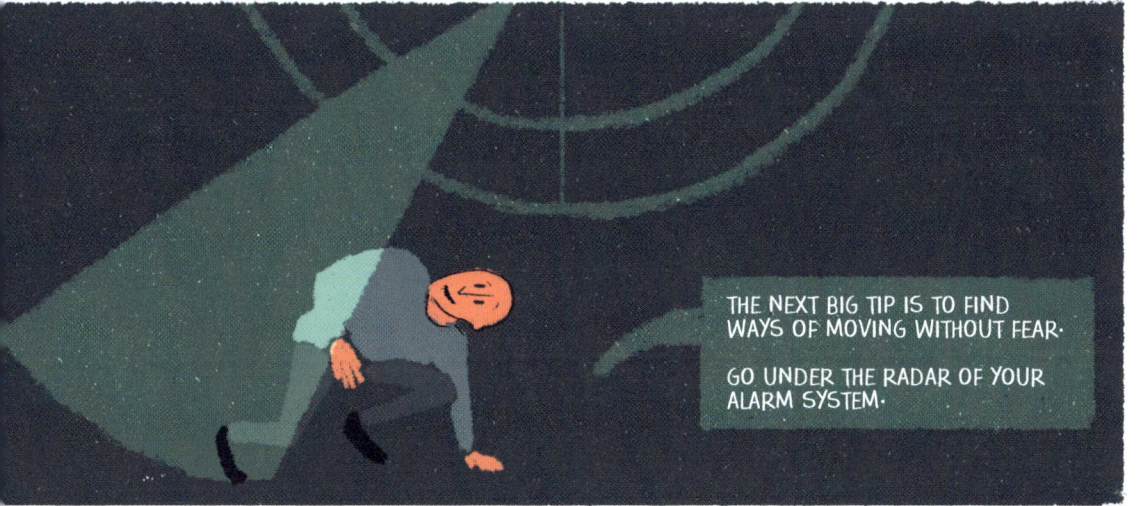

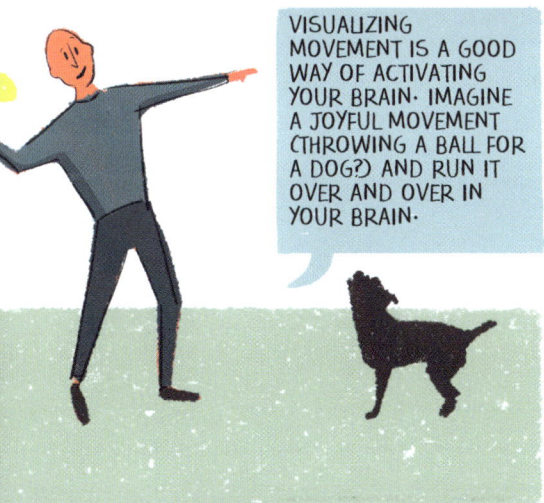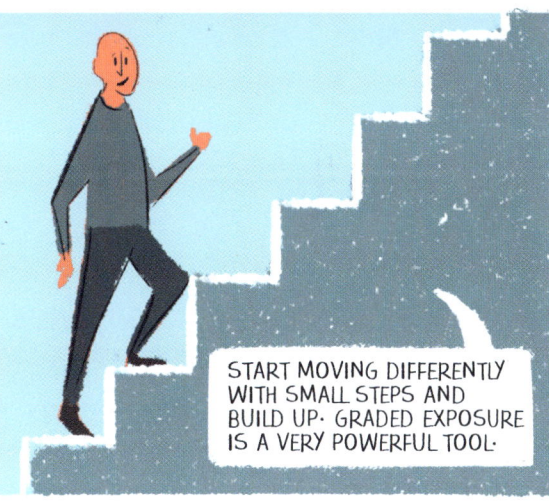

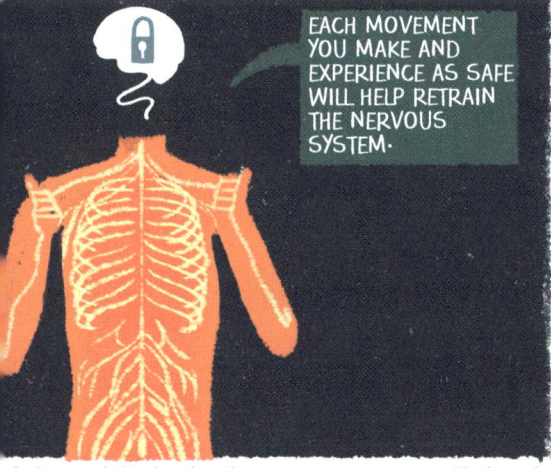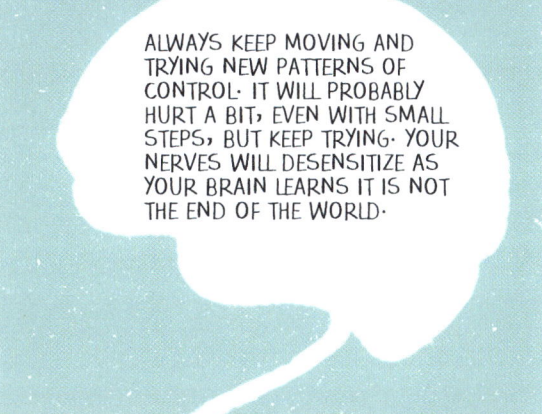

feelings and the thoughts about movement are inseparable from the ement itself' (Merzenich 2012). 'Graded exposure often involves using ivity to find alternative ways to painlessly perform a movement that is ally painful.' 'It gives the brain good news' (Hargrove 2014).

'We don't know which exercise programmes are best, but almost everything we try is getting them moving. It is important that the programmes contain education to reconceptualise pain as protective, and that the participants have a strong message that they are not broken' (Rovner 2014, World Congress on Pain).

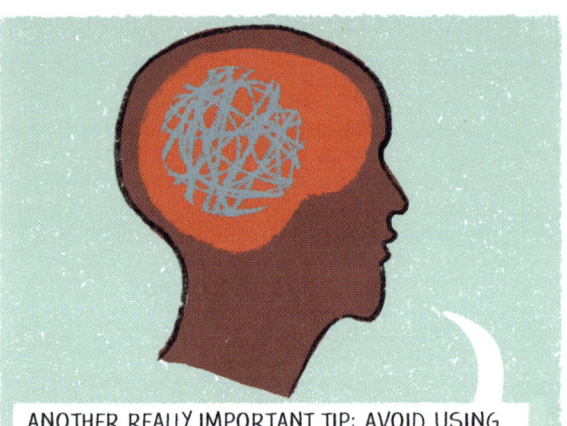

ANOTHER REALLY IMPORTANT TIP: AVOID USING LANGUAGE THAT MESSES WITH YOUR BRAIN. YOU CAN CHANGE THE PAIN NEUROTAG WITH NEW LANGUAGE AND CONCEPTS.

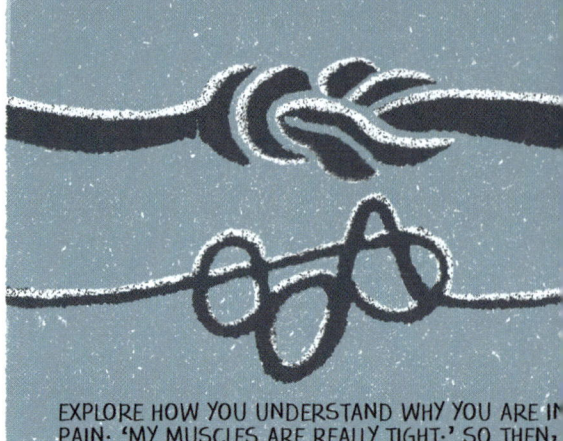

EXPLORE HOW YOU UNDERSTAND WHY YOU ARE IN PAIN. 'MY MUSCLES ARE REALLY TIGHT.' SO THEN, WHAT IS THE EXACT OPPOSITE OF TIGHT FOR YOU?

AN EXAMPLE OF UNHELPFUL LANGUAGE IS 'SLIPPED DISCS'. THEY SOUND SCARY, BUT THEY CAN NEVER HAPPEN. MAYBE USE THE METAPHOR OF A DISC UNDER PRESSURE OR SOMETHING BEING SQUEEZED, AND THEN FOCUS ON REDUCING THE PRESSURE AND HOW TO UNSQUEEZE.

MUCH LESS SCARY.

ANYTHING THAT DE-THREATENS THE SENSATIONS YOU ARE FEELING AND SUPPORTS NEW POSSIBILITIES WILL HELP BREAK THE PAIN HABIT. SELL YOURSELF MORE BEAUTIFUL, ELEGANT AND ACCURATE STORIES.

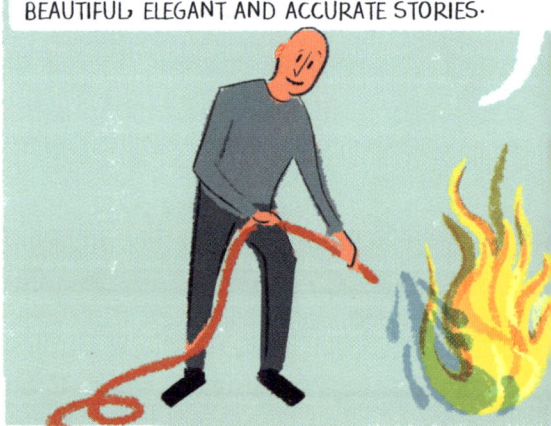

PLAY WITH METAPHORS THAT FIT YOU BUT OFFER THE POSSIBILITY OF CHANGE. AVOID PAIN AS AN EXTERNAL THING, PAIN AS VIOLENCE AND DAMAGE, PAIN AS YOUR FAULT (YOU DO NOT DESERVE TO SUFFER!) OR PAIN AS A BATTLE. THESE METAPHORS RARELY HELP.

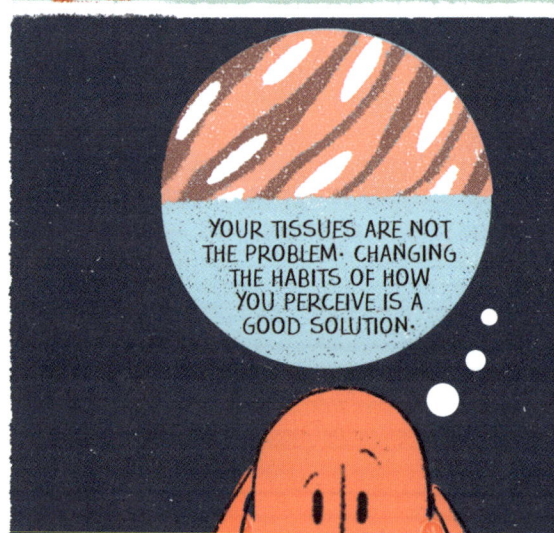

YOUR TISSUES ARE NOT THE PROBLEM. CHANGING THE HABITS OF HOW YOU PERCEIVE IS A GOOD SOLUTION.

If you've ever seen a disc in a cadaver you can't slip the suckers, they're immobile, but that's our language and it messes with your brain' (Moseley 2014).

Sciatica patients recovered about equally well with or without disc hernia visible on MRI scans in a large study in the New England Journal of Med (el Barzouhi et al 2013).

THINK OF CHANGING PAIN AS LEARNING TO WRITE WITH YOUR...
OPPOSITE HAND
HOW DO YOU CHANGE MEMORIES? HOW DO YOU CHANGE BELIEF SYSTEMS?
HOW DO YOU CHANGE HABITS AND REFLEXES?
LOTS OF THINGS ARE INVOLVED AND IT NEEDS WORK AND EXPERIMENTATION. BUT ALL THESE THINGS ARE MALLEABLE.
PAIN
PAIN
EMBER PAIN O MUCH E THAN BLEMS IN TISSUES BLOCKED TIONS.
CHRONIC PAIN ALWAYS INVOLVES A SENSITIZED NERVOUS SYSTEM.
A COMPLEX PROBLEM BENEFITS FROM A MULTITUDE OF CREATIVE RESPONSES. EVERYTHING ABOUT YOU IS RELEVANT.

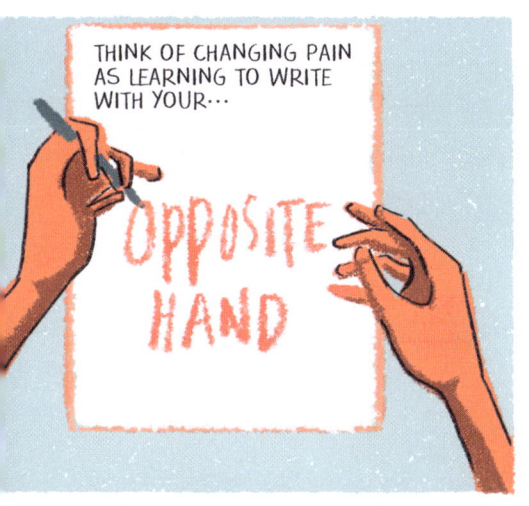

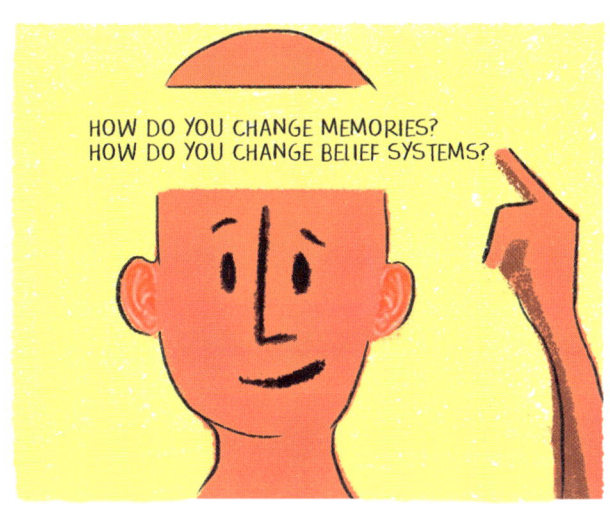

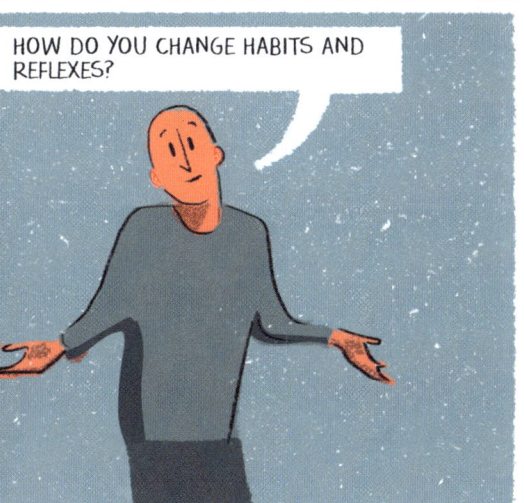

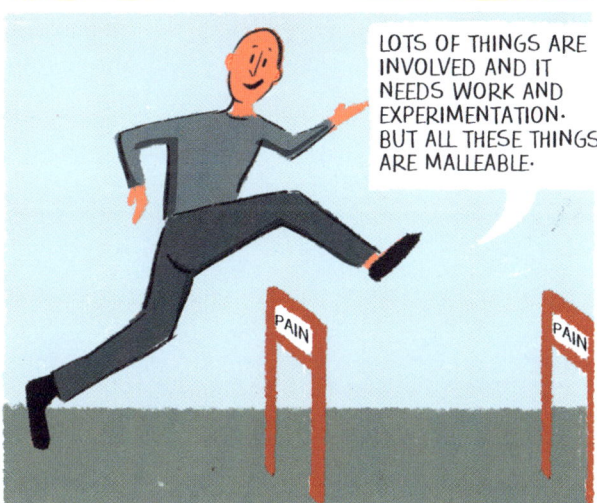

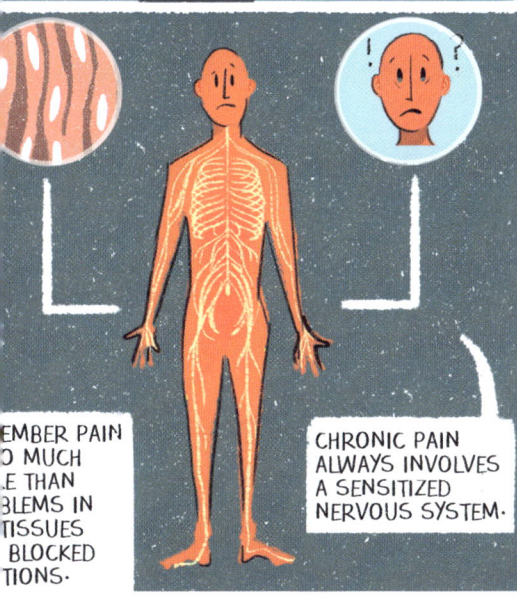

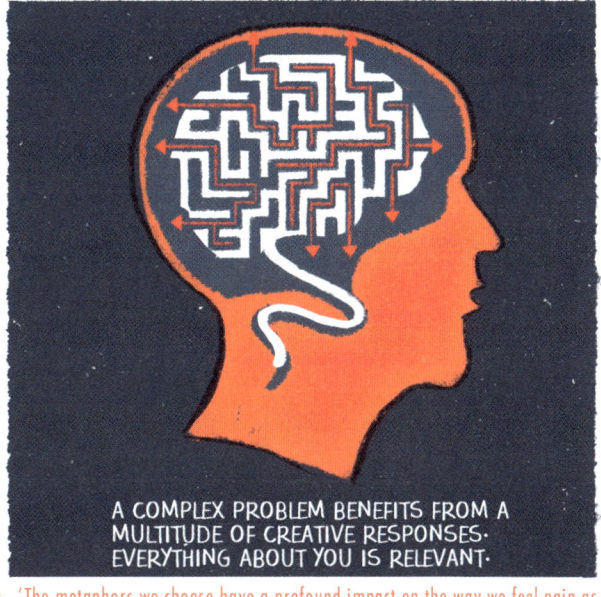

ding pain theorist David Butler, co-author of the hugely influential book Pain, changing metaphors is a central tool in changing the pain ence (Butler 2013).

'The metaphors we choose have a profound impact on the way we feel pain as well as upon the ways our suffering is treated' (Bourke 2014).

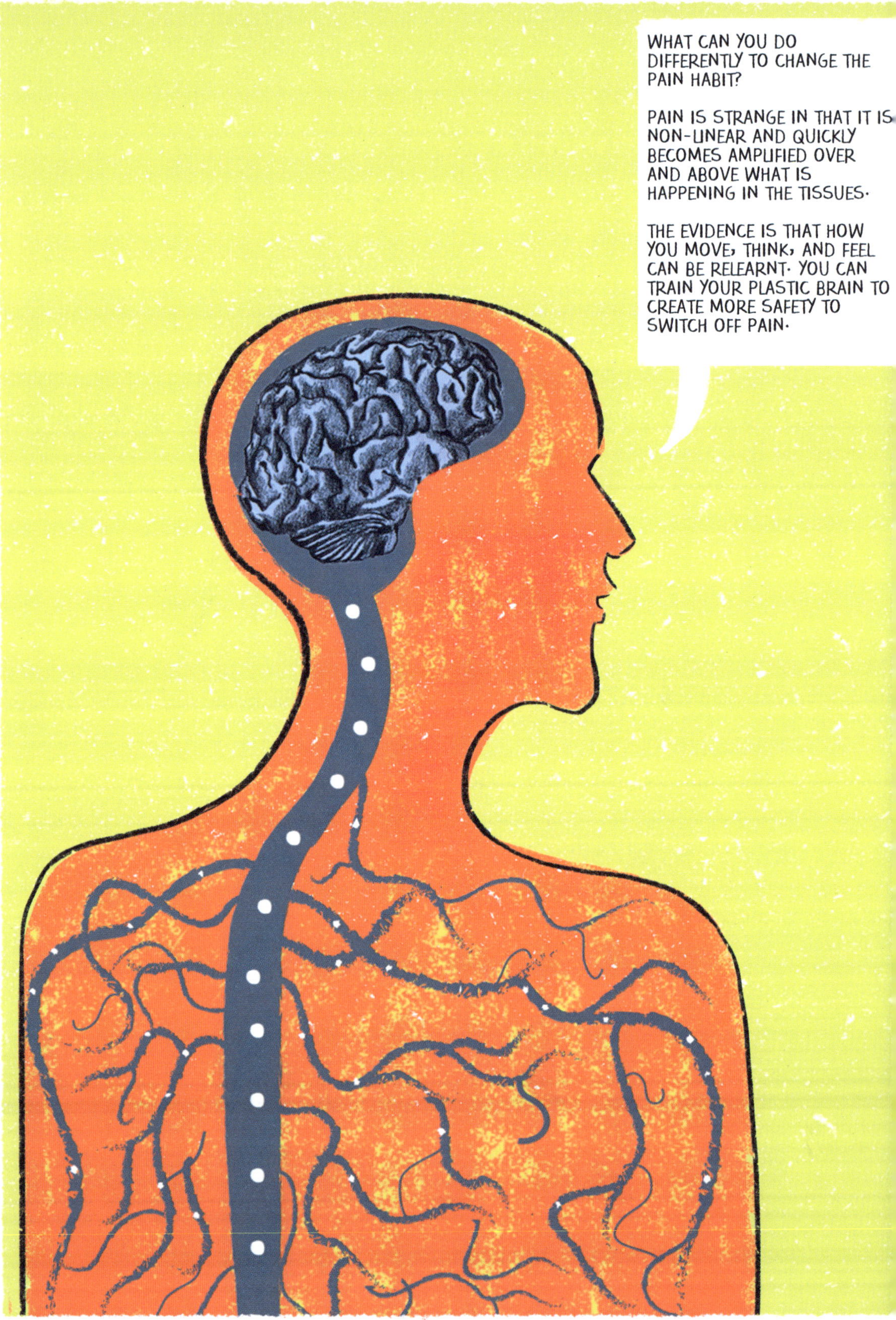
WHAT CAN YOU DO DIFFERENTLY TO CHANGE THE PAIN HABIT?
PAIN IS STRANGE IN THAT IT IS NON-LINEAR AND QUICKLY BECOMES AMPLIFIED OVER AND ABOVE WHAT IS HAPPENING IN THE TISSUES.
THE EVIDENCE IS THAT HOW YOU MOVE, THINK, AND FEEL CAN BE RELEARNT. YOU CAN TRAIN YOUR PLASTIC BRAIN TO CREATE MORE SAFETY TO SWITCH OFF PAIN.